OXFORD MEDICAL PUBLICATIONS

Clinical Dermatology

Oxford Core Texts

CLINICAL DERMATOLOGY

CLINICAL DERMATOLOGY

Rona M. MacKie

Professor of Dermatology
University of Glasgow;
Consultant Dermatologist,
Greater Glasgow Health Board,
West Glasgow University NHS Trust,
Yorkhill Children's Hospital NHS Trust

FOURTH EDITION

Oxford   New York   Toronto
Oxford University Press
1997

Oxford University Press, Walton Street, Oxford OX2 6DP

Oxford New York
Athens Auckland Bangkok Bombay
Calcutta Cape Town Dar es Salaam Delhi
Florence Hong Kong Istanbul Karachi
Kuala Lumpur Madras Madrid Melbourne
Mexico City Nairobi Paris Singapore
Taipei Tokyo Toronto
and associated companies in
Berlin Ibadan

Oxford is a trade mark of Oxford University Press

Published in the United States
by Oxford University Press Inc., New York

A catalogue record for this book is available from the British Library

Library of Congress Cataloging-in-Publication Data
MacKie, Rona M.
    Clinical dermatology / Rona M. MacKie.—4th ed.
        p.   cm.—(Oxford core texts) (Oxford medical publications)
    Includes bibliographical references and index.
    ISBN 0–19–262763–5 (hbk)   ISBN 0–19–2627619 (pbk)
    I. Title.   II. Series   III. Series: Oxford medical publications.
    [DNLM: 1. Skin Diseases.   WR 140 M158c 1996]
    RL71.M254   1996
    616.5–dc20
    DNLM/DLC
    for Library of Congress   96–12366
                                                                CIP

Typeset by
EXPO Holdings, Malaysia

Printed in Hong Kong

Preface

In preparing the fourth edition of this textbook, I have taken into consideration the increased and welcome move to small-group teaching, often in a community setting. It has been assumed that in many situations, undergraduates, residents, and other postgraduates will be given guidance and references, but be expected to work relatively independently. I have also assumed that in many parts of the world, teachers find their lives busier and that time for teaching is competing even more than in the past with clinical and administrative commitments.

This edition of the textbook has, therefore, undergone major revision both in terms of content and layout. In addition to providing a sound foundation of clinical dermatology with a substantial increase in illustrations, individual case problems have been introduced into the beginning of each chapter, with suggested diagnoses and management plans at the end. It is hoped that these will encourage active learning and also stimulate group discussion. All the information necessary to make a reasonable response to each of these problems will be found in the text of the relevant chapter, but at the end of a proportion of these problems, further questions are asked which may require a literature search outwith this book.

I have also included suggested project work at the end of each chapter and hope that some of these projects will be the starting point for dissertations and mini-theses in the newer medical curricula. These projects will be more productive if the reader has access either to online databases or to CD Rom reference discs. Sources of such data include the American Academy of Dermatology's Derminfonet, Medline, ISI BIDS, and others which should be readily available in a teaching hospital or University library, or personally by modem through the British Medical Association. If none of these is available, a session in a good library will, I hope, be stimulating and rewarding.

Thus, this book has been redesigned to be used as part of a learning package interacting with new information technologies. I hope that the end result will be a more enjoyable, thought provoking, and permanent learning experience.

I am grateful to my patients, both past and present, who form the basis of the case presentations throughout the book, and also to Mrs Pamela Sutherland for assistance with word processing.

Glasgow   R.M.M.
June 1996

Contents

1

Dermatological disability: incidence, prevalence, and classification of skin disease

Introduction

The skin is one of the largest organs in the body. Table 1.1 lists some of its important functions. These include protection from external injury, control of fluid balance and electrolytes, temperature control, an important outpost of the nervous system, an important outpost of the immune system, absorption of (and response to) ultraviolet radiation by synthesizing Vitamin D, and lipid synthesis. In addition to all this, the skin has an important cosmetic function.

From the list itemized in Table 1.1, it will be no surprise to read that around 10 per cent of consultations in primary care in the UK concern a dermatological disorder. What is not yet well known is the level of unmet need in the community. These are individuals who have chosen to live with their chronic psoriasis, recurrent hand dermatitis, or other problems either because they have in the past sought help and been unsatisfied with the response from the medical profession, or because they are not aware that anything can be done for their problem. There have been fairly rapid advances in the control, if not cure, of many skin diseases in the past 20 years. For example the ranges of treatments available for psoriasis and acne, both common skin diseases, are now much wider than 10 years ago. Nowadays, no teenager should end up with scarring as a result of acne lesions.

In addition to those individuals in the community who do not seek conventional medical help, there will be a further section of the dermatologically disabled who may seek help from practitioners of alternative or unorthodox medicine. These treatments should be assessed, if possible, in the same manner as are treatments used in conventional medicine so that patients can be given facts on comparative response rates and toxicity to help them participate in informed choices about their individual treatment plans.

Key Points

> Dermatological disorders account for 10 per cent of primary care consultations. In addition, there is considerable unmet need in the community, though this is difficult to quantify.

Table 1.1.
Important functional properties of the skin

Protects from external injury
Literally holds all other organs together
Plays a part in fluid balance. Mainly excretes but can also absorb fluid
Temperature control
An important organ of sensation
Absorbs ultraviolet radiation
Metabolizes vitamin D
Synthesizes epidermal lipids which are an important protective barrier
Cosmetic function

Dermatological disability

The quantity of physical and psychological disability which this unmet need for dermatological care causes cannot be estimated but must be considerable. Even

Key Points

To achieve a better assessment of the impact of skin disease, dermatological disability indices have been designed.

when the more severe skin diseases such as epidermolysis bullosa are reviewed (p. 237), any attempt to carry out a community-based survey of prevalence reveals many previously unrecognized sufferers. It is therefore assumed that this unmet need may be considerably greater in commoner but less severe problems.

Quantitating dermatological disability is not straightforward. However, in the past 5 years attempts to produce series of questions which will help measure the size of the problem have been devised. For example the psoriasis disability index (p. 53) is a series of simple questions which have been derived after talking to large numbers of patients with psoriasis and are designed to identify the level of disruption caused by the patient's skin problem with regard to certain aspects of life including domestic life, employment, and social activities. It may be instructive to you, and useful for the patient, to ask these questions both before and after a course of treatment to see whether or not **your** assessment of the value of your chosen treatment coincides with the patient's views. Remember also that dermatological disability may effect a whole family not just the patient. This is very obvious in the case of children with atopic eczema. The affected child may keep the whole family awake at night and take up a large proportion of his or her mother's time by day as she applies ointments, bandages the child, and tries to distract him from persistent scratching which will give rise to further problems.

The size of the problem

Dermatological diseases can be measured by their incidence and prevalence. The incidence of any disease is the number of new cases identified over a period of time, usually a calendar year. A striking example of the rising incidence of a particular skin disease is the situation with cutaneous malignant melanoma where the incidence is currently doubling every 10 years, a rate of increase faster than for any other type of cancer except lung cancer in women.

The prevalence of a disease is the term used to describe the numbers of cases of any condition in the population at a given time. Thus, long-lasting chronic conditions such as psoriasis or eczema are likely to have a high prevalence, whereas conditions which tend to affect individuals for only a short period of time and either burn out or cause the patient's death will have a lower prevalence. Over the past 20 years, the prevalence of atopic disorders—asthma, allergic rhinitis, and atopic eczema—have all increased steeply for reasons which are not yet entirely understood.

Table 1.2 lists the main conditions currently contributing to the workload of a hospital dermatology department. This is the list of the ten conditions most commonly referred over the period 1992–1994 to a major European teaching hospital. By comparison with referrals 10 years previously, there is a rapidly rising dermatological workload in the field of cutaneous malignancy and possible pre-cancerous lesions. Whereas 10 years ago a higher proportion of patients were referred with inflammatory skin diseases such as dermatitis and acne, the tendency to refer patients with potentially malignant lesions has grown steadily. This may either reflect a desire on the part of the general practitioner for a

Table 1.2.

The commonest causes for dermatological referral to a northern European teaching hospital 1992–1994

Psoriasis

Acne

Dermatitis

Seborrhoeic keratoses

Basal cell carcinoma

Actinic keratosis

Alopecia areata

Fungal infections

Melanocytic naevi

Warts

Key Points

Numbers of cases of a disease are measured by their incidence (number of new cases identified in a time period) and prevalence (number of cases in a population at a given time).

second opinion concerning this potentially serious group of malignant or pre-malignant skin diseases or a genuine increase in their numbers in the community.

Classification of skin disease

There is no entirely satisfactory method of classification of skin diseases. Traditionally dermatologists have used a morphological classification where the condition was described, often in Latin. At the present time, modern dermatologists are doing their best to describe skin disease according to biochemically defined functional or genetic abnormalities. This is proceeding slowly but there are still areas where the old and the new terminology do not quite equate. Thus, it would be logical to assume that all skin diseases called epidermolysis bullosa were associated with **blisters** and **lysis** of cells in the epidermis. In fact only one subset of the epidermolysis bullosa collection of disorders does have these characteristics, and some of the others have clearly identified abnormalities of collagen genes or of keratin genes. Some rethinking and renaming of morphologically inaccurately described diseases is now feasible thanks to recent scientific advances.

A further method of thinking about skin disease in terms of classification is to consider the various ages of life at which the diseases are most prevalent. Thus, a chronological classification can divide the speciality into paediatric, adolescent, adult, and geriatric dermatology with perhaps a subset of occupational dermatology for those in employment. This is not entirely satisfactory as although some conditions such as angiomas and atopic dermatitis are very much commoner in early infancy, they may continue to be problems throughout life. Thus, although the paediatric dermatology can be a recognized but fairly specialized subdivision of dermatology, it is necessary for those who practise paediatric dermatology to be fully trained dermatologists with a knowledge of adult disease as well. Clearly, it is highly desirable if they are also fully trained paediatricians. Similar caveats apply to chronological classifications at the other end of the age spectrum where geriatric dermatology requires a knowledge of the whole of dermatology and also of the care and management of the elderly.

A brief glossary of useful clinical and histological terms follows to help in both spoken and written communication.

Acantholysis: a rounding up of epidermal cells resulting from a loss of adhesion between these cells. Seen in association with benign blistering disease (pemphigus) and in epidermal malignancy.

Acanthosis: histological term used to describe epidermal thickening due to an increase in the number of cells in the prickle cell layer.

Atopy: Literally 'strange disease'. The triad of atopic dermatitis, asthma, and allergic rhinitis (hay fever).

Balloon degeneration: gross swelling of keratinocytes in epidermal viral infection. Both the nucleus and cytoplasm are affected.

Basement membrane: a multi-layered structure between epidermis and dermis.

Bowen's carcinoma *in situ* (**Bowen's disease**): a form of intraepidermal carcinoma *in situ* characterized by the presence of atypical giant cells with aberrant mitotic figures.

Cheiropompholyx: an eruption of the sides of the fingers and palms of the hands composed of multiple small blisters.

Civatte bodies (colloid bodies): amorphous pink globules seen at the dermo-epidermal junction in certain diseases characterized by damage to and death of basal cells (for example lichen planus).

Comedo (blackhead): a plug of oxidized sebaceous material obstructing the surface opening of pilosebaceous follicle.

Desmosomes: specialized areas of intraepidermal adhesion between keratinocytes.

Dyskeratosis: premature and atypical keratinization of epidermal cells.

Ecthyma: a pyogenic skin infection characterized by superficial crusting and underlying ulceration.

Ephelis (freckle): a localized area of increased pigment synthesis by melanocytes.

Hirsuties: excessive growth of male-pattern hair.

Hyperkeratosis: excessive formation of normal keratin for the body site in question.

Hypertrichosis: excessive growth of non-androgen dependent hair.

Ichthyosis ('fish skin'): excessively dry and scaly skin.

Inclusion bodies: eosinophilic bodies with a clear surrounding halo. Seen in cutaneous viral infections.

Intertrigo: dermatitis on apposing areas of skin in flexural body sites (groins, axillae).

Kerion: a severe pustular reaction on the scalp in children. Caused by animal ringworm.

Lichenification: thickening (acanthosis) of the epidermis resulting in accentuation of normal skin markings.

Liquefaction degeneration: damage to the epidermal basal layer, seen principally in lichen planus and lupus erythematosus.

Miliaria: vesicular lesions resulting from occlusion of eccrine sweat ducts. Common in hot, humid environments.

Nikolsky's sign: the shearing of epidermis from dermis produced by lateral pressure on the epidermal surface. Positive in pemphigus vulgaris.

Parakeratosis: abnormal or incomplete keratinization resulting in the presence of nucleated, flattened squamous cells in the stratum corneum.

Reticular degeneration (*see also* **balloon degeneration**): an intraepidermal blister resulting from balloon degenerations of virally infected epidermal cells. Some cell walls are retained and the blister thus has a multiloculated reticular framework.

Rhinophyma: gross hypertrophy of sebaceous gland tissue resulting in increase in volume of nasal soft tissue. A complication of rosacea.

Spongiosis: oedema of the epidermis, mainly intracellular.

Wickham's striae: white linear markings on the surface of the violaceous papules of lichen planus.

Projects

1. Ask the centre in which you are working (hospital, health centre, general practice, or other setting) for the disease index relating to dermatological attendances and referrals over the last 6 to 12 months. Do you think that the conditions which have been diagnosed in the setting in which you are currently working reflect either the prevalence or the incidence of these conditions in the community? If not, why not? Do you think the numbers of patients seen and their diagnoses relates to severity of the disease, desire to improve employment prospects, or desire to improve cosmetic appearance? What other reasons might prompt patients to seek treatment for a chronic skin condition ?

2. How could you go about substantiating the hypothesis that patients seeking help for dermatological problems do not accurately reflect the proportion of these specific dermatological diseases in a community at large?

3. If you were asked to provide a blueprint for dermatological care in the setting in which you are currently working in the year 2001, which conditions would you predict would have increased in incidence and or prevalence and why? Similarly, which conditions would you hope and anticipate would have become less of a problem? Could you make your task more likely to be accurate by studying models of care elsewhere in the world? If yes, give details.

2

Essential skin biology: structure, function, and immunology

- Anatomy of the normal skin

The skin is a large and complex structure. An understanding of basic structure and function should help make your approach to skin disease more logical, and also increase your interest in the skin as a major organ of the body.

Anatomy of the normal skin

The skin can be divided into three main functional areas. These are the:

- **epidermis**   the major protective layer derived from the fetal ectoderm;

- **dermis**   the major support layer—of mesodermal origin;

- **skin appendages** composed of cells derived from both ectoderm and mesoderm

>   hair follicle
>
>   sebaceous gland
>
>   apocrine sweat gland
>
>   eccrine sweat gland
>
>   nails.

- In addition a fourth area, the subcutaneous **fat**, may be involved in deeply situated skin lesions such as erythema nodosum (p. 177).

The epidermis

Beginning at the outer surface and working inwards, four clear layers of epidermis can be observed using the light microscope (Fig. 2.1). These are the:

- **cornified or horny layer**   outer non-nucleated barrier layer;

- **granular layer**   the zone where epidermal nuclei disintegrate;

Key Points

The epidermis consists of four layers—the cornified layer (an outer, non-nucleated barrier), granular (nuclei disintegrating), germinative or prickle cell (bulk of living keratinocytes), and basal layer (normally the only site of epidermal mitosis).

Fig. 2.1 Skin from palm of hand. The cornified layer (c), the granular layer (g), and the keratinocytes in the germinative layer (k) are all easily seen.

- germinative or prickle cell layer   the bulk of the living epidermal keratinocytes;

- basal layer   the only keratinocytes in **normal** epidermis which undergo cell division.

These layers are best seen if a piece of thick, weight-bearing skin, such as that from the sole of the foot, is examined under the microscope. In this thick skin, a fifth layer can sometimes be seen just above the granular layer—the **stratum lucidum.** It is not certain whether or not this is really a functionally distinct layer or an artefact of preparation.

It is useful to become familiar with the appearance of normal skin by using the microscope to examine areas at the normal margins of excision biopsies to build up experience of the normal physiological variations in appearance of healthy skin in different body sites at different ages. For example non-weight-bearing skin, such as that on the inner upper arm, has a thin cornified layer and only three or four underlying layers of keratinocytes whereas the keratinocyte layer of the sole of the foot is 20–30 cells thick. On chronically sun-exposed sites, chiefly the face, both the epidermis and the underlying dermis may show very marked changes due to accumulated exposure to natural sunlight. This is photoageing and is seen clinically as thickened, wrinkled, furrowed yellowish skin. Many of the alterations in the skin which we think of as ageing are in fact due to UV-induced damage, and distinction should be made between **photoageing,** which is at least partially preventable, and chronological or **biological** ageing. Figures 2.2 and 2.3 show the exposed facial skin and non-exposed trunk skin of the same 84-year-old to emphasize this point.

Cell types seen in the epidermis

These are the:

- keratinocyte   the main cell type;

- melanocyte   found in the basal layer, the pigment-producing cell;

- Langerhans cell   found in the mid-dermis—an important immunologically competent cell;

- Merkel cell   found in and around the basal layer. A member of the amine precursor uptake and decarboxylation (APUD) system.

The keratinocyte

The keratinocyte forms the great bulk of the cells in the epidermis. In normal skin, keratinocyte division takes place only in the basal layer, so mitotic figures should not normally be seen above this level. After cell division, one daughter keratinocyte remains in the basal layer and the other moves upwards through the epidermis. This keratinocyte is committed to terminal differentiation and death. Within the prickle cell layer, the keratinocytes are connected to each other by highly specialized cellular bridges, called **desmosomes,** and these can frequently be seen under the light microscope at high power. They may be particularly easy to see in a biopsy from early dermatitis where there is a lot of

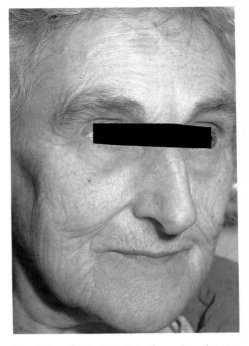

epidermal oedema (Fig. 2.4). There are no desmosomes between keratinocytes and melanocytes, or Langerhans cells, or Merkel cells. There are hemi-desmosomes between the basal layer keratinocytes and the underlying basement membrane.

In the **granular layer**, (Fig. 2.5) the living keratinocytes are involved in a complex series of biochemical changes during which the cell nuclei disintegrate, forming the granules seen in the cytoplasm. Above this level there is the non-nucleated stratum corneum, or cornified layer.

Development and maturation of normal healthy epidermis in this pattern is called orthokeratosis, and produces an outer layer of non-nucleated, dead, flat keratinocytes. In some mucosal sites the normal maturation pattern is different,

Figs 2.2 and 2.3 Skin of the face and trunk on an 84-year-old female who has lived all her life in Scotland. The wrinkling and pigment variation of the chronically exposed facial skin are not seen on the normally covered skin. The contrast would be much greater had she lived in a sunnier climate such as Australia.

Fig. 2.4 Skin biopsy from a patient with contact dermatitis in the early acute state. There is a lot of oedema in the epidermis, and this shows the desmosomes stretched between adjacent keratinocytes (arrow). In some cases the desmosemes have become ruptured.

Fig. 2.5 High-power view of granular layer, showing sharp transition from the living but non-dividing epidermal cells and the dead anucleate cornified layer.

Key Points

Normal development of keratinocytes is orthokeratosis. In some mucosal sites physiological parakeratosis occurs.

and there is no granular layer, but an outer layer of nucleated squamous cells. The term for this pattern is **physiological parakeratosis** (Fig. 2.6).

Pathological parakeratosis is seen in some diseases of the epidermis, psoriasis being the most common example. In this situation the normal differentiation signals are either lacking or overridden and there is accelerated and imperfect development of the stratum corneum. If keratinocytes are grown in tissue culture, they will come together and form interconnecting desmosomes, but the outer layer is parakeratotic as in psoriasis rather than orthokeratototic as in normal skin.

It is calculated that the 'transit time' for a daughter keratinocyte in the basal layer of normal skin to reach the outer surface is around 50–75 days. In psoriasis this is reduced to 8–10 days.

Fig. 2.6 Mucous membrane showing normal physiological parakeratosis seen in this site. Nuclei are present in the upper layers and thus there is no granular layer.

The strength of the epidermis depends on the cohesion of the keratinocytes. They produce a structural protein, alpha-keratin, which aggregates to form tonofilaments. These tonofilaments are continuous with the desmosomes and are easily seen in the electron microscope as large cytoplasmic bundles. Another communication channel between keratinocytes are gap junctions, tiny channels which connect the cytoplasm of neighbouring cells to each other.

Genetic abnormalities of keratinization and resulting disease states

Keratins are synthesized by the keratinocytes in pairs, one basic and one acidic keratin. The basal layer of the epidermis synthesizes keratins 5 and 14, and genetic disturbances in the genes coding for these keratins causes the disease epidermolysis bullosa simplex (p. 238); while the suprabasal keratinocytes synthesize keratins 1 and 10, and abnormalities give rise to bullous ichthyosiform erythroderma or epidermolytic hyperkeratosis (p. 70). Exact gene mapping of other disorders of keratinization is in progress.

Cell adhesion molecules

Cell adhesion and the molecules which facilitate it are of great importance in all tissues. Intercellular Adhesion Molecule (ICAM) is expressed on the surface of keratinocytes and forms one half of a 'lock and key' arrangement between these keratinocytes and lymphocytes, which traffic in small numbers through the epidermis and express Lymphocyte Function Antigen (LFA) on their surface. Thus the ICAM molecule on the surface of the keratinocyte links physically with LFA expressed on the lymphocyte surface, and subsequently triggers lymphokine release in conditions such as dermatitis (p. 78).

Integrins

The integrin family are another group of important cell surface proteins associated with adhesion. LFA is a member of this family, and different integrins are characterized by expression of a wide range of alpha and beta chains. Alpha-6-beta-4-integrin appears to be particularly important in adhesion of the basal cells to the basement membrane, and thus it is of potential importance in diseases characterized by blisters at this level, such as bullous pemphigoid (p. 233).

Cadherins

The cadherin family of adhesion molecules play a major part in adhesion of suprabasal keratinocytes to each other in association with the desmosomes. Desmoglein is a member of this family, and faulty adhesion between keratinocytes due to abnormalities of these molecules is associated with the pemphigus group of blistering disorders (p. 229).

Cells expressing MHC class 2 antigens

In the normal epidermis, the only cells which normally express the MHC class 2 antigens HLA-DR, -DP, and -DQ are the Langerhans cells (see below). In a wide range of skin diseases, MHC class 2 molecule expression is induced on keratinocytes. HLA-DR, HLA-DP and HLA-DQ expression are all markers of immunologically activated and competent cells, indicating that in appropriate circumstances the keratinocytes can actively contribute to immunological reactions, not just respond as innocent bystanders.

The melanocyte

Pigment production in the skin is an important function of the epidermal melanocyte. These cells can be seen with H & E staining as small cells in the basal layer, often with a clear halo around them, presumably because of the absence of desmosomes holding them to adjacent basal keratinocytes. In Fig. 2.7 a silver stain has been used to show that melanocytes have multiple dendrites and these dendritic processes stretch between adjacent keratinocytes, bringing melanocytes into surface contact with a relatively large number of keratinocytes. On facial skin there may be as many as one melanocyte for every five basal layer keratinocytes, but in the lower back skin this ratio is usually closer to one in 20. Chronic light exposure increases the number of melanocytes relative to keratinocytes, so that there are more in the skin of the outer upper arm than in the skin of the inner upper arm. Numbers of melanocytes are the same in equivalent body sites in white and black skin, but the rate of production of pigment and its distribution is different. Darker skinned races have more active melanocytes, and distribute melanin pigment to surrounding keratinocytes in smaller packages than is the case in paler skinned individuals.

Melanocytes synthesize the pigment melanin. Melanin granules are seen on ultrastructural examination as small, black, electron-dense, intracytoplasmic structures—the melanosomes. The pigment is formed from DOPA on pre-melanosomes and this biochemical reaction is catalysed by the presence in the melanocyte of the enzymes dopa-oxidase and tyrosinase, which are not present in surrounding keratinocytes or other non-melanocytic cells.

Fig. 2.7 Melanocytes in the epidermis stained with silver. Note the dendritic shape of the cells.

Once the melanin granules are formed, they are distributed along the dendrites of the melanocytes and from there to surrounding keratinocytes. The combination of one pigment-producing melanocyte and several surrounding keratinocytes receiving melanin granules is termed the 'epidermal melanin unit'. Thus, the presence of melanin in a cell does not prove that cell to be a melanocyte and specific biochemical evidence that the cell actually produces melanin is needed, by demonstrating that the cell in question contains the enzyme tyrosinase.

Melanocytes are found in man in greatest quantities in the epidermis, the hair bulb, the eye, the brain, and in very small numbers in other organs. Their function in normal skin is thought to be to provide protection from ultraviolet radiation. This appears to be reasonably effective in that sunlight-induced skin cancers of all types are much rarer on black skin than on white skin.

The Langerhans cell

This cell was discovered in 1860 by Paul Langerhans when he was a medical student, and until the 1960s it had no clearly defined function. In the last 30 years there has been a dramatic advance in our knowledge of this cell which is now recognized as an important immunologically competent cell. The Langerhans cell is derived from the bone marrow and is found on all epidermal surfaces, usually in the middle area of the epidermis. On H & E stained sections, the Langerhans cell may be seen as a slightly larger cell than those around it, with a clear halo, possibly due, as with the melanocyte, to the lack of desmosomes. To see the Langerhans cell clearly, immunocytochemistry is necessary using one of the antibodies which recognizes Langerhans cells either on formalin-fixed, paraffin-processed material (for example antibody to S100) or on fresh frozen tissue (for example antibody to CD1). With this approach it will be seen that the Langerhans cell is a dendritic cell and that in most body sites it is

Key Points

Melanin is synthesized by melanocytes and moved to surrounding keratinocytes, and thus these cell types should be distinguished biochemically, not by presence of the pigment.

Fig. 2.8 Horizontal 'spread preparation' of the epidermis stained with an antibody specific for Langerhans cells. Note how the cells come into contact with each other by their dendritic processes and form a network.

Key Points

Langerhans cells are immunologically competent and may act as antigen presenting cells.

present in the epidermis in relatively large numbers, with the dendrites of one cell in close contact with those of the next (Fig. 2.8). The other approach to seeing this cell is to use the electron microscope. Langerhans cells are recognized at this magnification by the presence of highly specific intracytoplasmic structures, the Birbeck granules. These look rather like tennis or squash racquets (Fig. 2.9) and their function is not yet understood.

Langerhans cells in normal skin are the only cells to express MHC class 2 antigens and carry receptors for complement. They are currently believed to be members of the family of immunologically important dendritic cells found in a number of body sites including the lymph nodes and spleen. The immunological profile of these dendritic cells suggests that they have the capacity to act as antigen presenting cells. Antigen adheres very readily to their surface, but in contrast to classical macrophages, Langerhans cells do not phagocytose efficiently. In the epidermis, which obviously comes into contact with more foreign material than any other part of the body, this antigen-processing function may be of very great importance in, for example, allergic contact dermatitis—see p. 96.

Abnormal Langerhans cell proliferation is seen in a relatively rare proliferative condition, histiocytosis X (p. 299).

The Merkel cell

These cells at present require electron microscopy to be identified. Their cytoplasm is packed with electron dense granules, and the cells are found in large numbers in touch sensitive sites such as the fingertips and around the lips. They appear to be concentrated around the basement membrane area, and in association with nerve endings. Their granules contain large quantities of catecholamines, and because of this they are thought to be part of the APUD

Fig. 2.9 Ultrastructure of Langerhans cell, showing the characteristic and specific tennis racquet-shaped Birbeck granule in the cytoplasm.

(amine precursor uptake and decarboxylation) system. Their exact normal function is not known but is thought to be related to cutaneous sensation. A rare but aggressive tumour, the Merkel cell tumour, may arise from these cells, usually in sun damaged skin (p. 313).

The skin immune system

There is now unequivocal evidence that the skin is an immunologically competent organ. The individual components of this system can be called the skin immune system—SIS or skin associated lymphoid system—SALT. As the cells involved are more than just lymphocytes, SIS is more accurate. The SIS includes Langerhans cells , which can be considered modified macrophages, and part of the reticuloepithelial dendritic cell system, which is also found in organs such as the spleen and the lymph nodes. Lymphocytes may be seen trafficking through the epidermis and are most commonly T-lymphocytes, both of the TH1 and the TH2 subsets. In diseases such as graft-versus-host disease these lymphocytes may be seen in close apposition to necrotic keratinocytes which appears to be undergoing a type of programmed cell death described as apoptosis, and previously described as satellite cell necrosis.

Keratinocytes are also part of the cutaneous immune system in that they express MHC class 2 antigens when activated, and both secrete and respond to immunologically active cytokines. The subfamilies of cytokines include growth factors, the interleukin family and interferons.

Growth factors

A number of these are found in the epidermis and dermis in both healthy and diseased skin. Epidermal growth factor has a structure very similar to transforming growth factor alpha, and is synthesized by epidermal keratinocytes. Expression of TGF alpha is abnormal in psoriasis (p. 46). Transforming growth factor beta is also active in the skin and is associated with apparent over-activity of dermal fibroblasts in dermal hyperproliferative conditions such as keloid scarring and scleroderma. A further important growth factor is fibroblast growth factor which is a very important growth factor for normal melanocytes in culture and appears to be released in intact human skin after exposure to ultraviolet light. Thus, a number of growth factors do appear to play a part in maintaining normal cutaneous homeostasis. Their use in therapeutic situations in dermatology is at an earlier stage than is their use in haematological conditions, and carefully controlled randomized trials are needed to establish their place in dermatological therapy.

Interleukins

The family of interleukins is steadily increasing. At present 15 interleukins have been characterized. They are short-lived molecules and detection of interleukin mRNA, or the protein itself, in the epidermis is technically demanding. Nevertheless, it would appear for example that expression of IL-4 is abnormal in atopic dermatitis (p. 79).

Interferons

The interferon family comprise alpha, beta, and gamma interferons. Abnormal amounts of gamma interferon are seen in allergic contact dermatitis and is secreted from lymphocytes trafficking through the epidermis and possibly also by activated keratinocytes.

The basement membrane

The basement membrane divides the epidermis from the dermis, and is a complex multilayered structure. It is shown diagrammatically in Fig. 2.10 and ultrastructurally in Fig. 2.11. This shows that the basement membrane zone is a striking multilayered structure, and as different diseases result from abnormalities of each of these layers, some understanding of this area is of practical as well as academic interest. Hemidesmosomes attach the basal layer keratinocytes to the lamina lucida area. Hemidesmosome defects are seen in some variants of the genetically determined blistering disease epidermolysis bullosa, (p. 237) and

Fig. 2.10 Diagram of basement membrane zone to show its multilayered structure.

Fig. 2.11 Ultrastructure of basement membrane zone. Compare this with Fig. 2.10.

autoantibodies to components of the lamina lucida are found in the acquired autoimmune blistering disease, bullous pemphigoid (p. 233). Below this level is the subbasal dense plate through which anchoring filaments connect the lamina lucida to the lamina densa. This is an area which is rich in collagen type 4. Collagen type 7 is also found in this area, but situated a little deeper, and is deficient in the dystrophic type of epidermolysis bullosa.

In spite of the multiple layers of the basement membrane, it is not a rigid impervious structure but one through which cells such as lymphocytes and Langerhans cells can, and do, pass with relative ease. Also, the basement membrane is not a flat layer dividing epidermis above from dermis below like the filling in a sandwich, but is heavily convoluted, with most convolution being seen in areas of weight bearing skin, that is the soles of the feet. Here the dermal papillae, the superficial layer of the dermis, sticks up into the dermis like small pegs. These dermal papillae are also present, but less obvious, in thinner skinned sites; this is an arrangement which maximizes the surface area of contact between dermis and epidermis, and minimizes the chance of discohesion due to loss of contact between the two layers.

The dermis

The outer layer of the dermis is called the papillary dermis and contains finer collagen fibres than the deeper reticular dermis. This is easily seen if polarized light is used to examine sections of normal skin in the light microscope.

There are three main cell types in the dermis:

- the **fibroblast**   produces collagen;
- the **macrophage**   acts as a general scavenger;
- the **mast cell**   An important cell in type 1 immunological reactions and interactions with the eosinophil. May have additional functions.

The bulk of the dermis is composed of type 3 collagen, and running through this collagen there is a fine network of elastic fibres. Dermal proteoglycans surround this fibrous material and embedded within the dermis are the:

- **vasculature**
- **lymphatics**
- **nerves**
- small quantities of **smooth and striated muscle.**

The blood supply

The blood supply to both epidermis and dermis is through a very rich anastomosing superficial and deep plexus of small blood vessels. There is a very large overcapacity in the dermal vasculature which is normally only operating at 10–20 per cent of capacity. After vigorous physical exercise, heat loss via the skin is needed, and the vasculature dilates appropriately. In a number of skin diseases the blood supply to the skin is greatly increased, causing total body redness

Fig. 2.12 Injected post-mortem specimen showing the abundance of the dermal vasculature.

Fig. 2.13 Nerve endings demonstrated by a silver stain. Note the free nerve ending (f) and the encapsulated ending (e).

or erythroderma. The volume of blood flowing through the dilated dermal vessels in this situation can be so great that high-output cardiac failure can be induced. Figure 2.12 shows the profuse network of small vessels in the papillary dermis and the scattered larger, deeper vessels, with a network of vessels around skin appendages.

In normal skin the lymphatic drainage system is not visible, but this is also a profuse network, running from the reticular dermis to the local lymph nodes.

Cutaneous nerves

Both free nerve ending and specialized receptors will be seen in the dermis. These nerve endings are important for the sense of touch, heat, cold, and proprioception. Nerve endings are best seen on light microscopy with a silver stain, and are numerous in the papillary dermis (Fig. 2.13). Striking specialized receptors, the Pacinian and Meissner corpuscles are also present (Fig. 2.14).

The skin appendages

These are the pilosebaceous unit, the eccrine sweat glands, and the nails. The pilosebaceous unit includes the:

- **hair follicle**
- **sebaceous gland**
- **arrector pili muscle**

and in some sites, for example axilla, the

- **apocrine gland.**

The pilosebaceous unit is shown diagramatically in Fig. 2.15 and histologically in Fig. 2.16. On the scalp, the predominant structure is the hair follicle with the sebaceous gland seen as a small insignificant attachment. A small strip of smooth muscle, the arrector pili muscle, may be seen, often around a lobule of

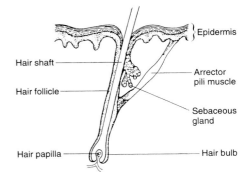

Fig. 2.14 Another type of nerve ending, the Pacinian corpuscle. This is responsible for the sensation of deep pressure.

Fig. 2.15 Diagram of the pilosebaceous unit.

Fig. 2.16 The pilosebaceous unit, showing the sebaceous gland draining into the hair follicle canal.

sebaceous gland, and in the axilla the apocrine glands may also be seen draining into the duct leading to the surface.

The **hair follicle** is the result of interaction between downgrowth of fetal ectoderm, which will form the hair shaft, and the vascular hair bulb papilla, which is derived from fetal mesoderm (Fig. 2.17).

The hair shaft itself is a complex multilayered structure with an outer cortex and an inner medulla. There are three recognizable types of hair. These are the coarse terminal hair of the scalp, the androgen-dependent terminal hair on the male chin, in the axilla, and the pubic region, and a fine growth of downy vellous hair on all body sites.

The control of growth of scalp hair is poorly understood. At any one time 80 per cent of scalp hair is growing in **anagen**, and the remaining 20 per cent is

Fig. 2.17 High-power view of hair root, showing the root of the hair derived from the epidermis stretched around the dermal papilla.

either resting—in **catagen**—or being shed—in **telogen** (Fig. 2.18). Normally, this programmed replacement of hair is scattered randomly over the scalp so that no single area is totally depleted at one time, but in **alopecia areata** (p. 212) all the hair in one scalp area is shed simultaneously.

The **sebaceous glands** are clusters of cells with a small dark nucleus and a foamy cytoplasm which are well illustrated in Fig. 2.16. They cluster around the hair shafts and their secretion is formed by total destruction of the cells, a mechanism called holocrine secretion. This secretion drains into the hair follicle and is discharged on the surface through the hair follicle opening. Sebaceous glands are seen in large numbers on the face, chest, and upper back. They may be obvious as small raised pearly nodules on the face of neonates, when their enlargement is due to carry-over of maternal hormones. They rapidly shrink and become vestigial until puberty when, in response to the individual's own hormones, they become large and active—sometimes overactive. This is the main cause of acne vulgaris (p. 205).

The **apocrine sweat glands** are found predominantly in the axilla, with a few seen also in the skin of the groin. They have a secretory component seen in the deeper dermis. This secretory section has a very wide lumen, and the cells lining this lumen will be seen to be composed of columnar epithelium which appears to form glandular secretion by a 'nipping off' of the tops of the cells, a process known as **decapitation secretion** (Figs 2.19 and 2.20). The excretory channels of the apocrine glands most commonly drain into the canal of the hair shaft and sebum passes from here out on to the surface of the epidermis.

The **eccrine sweat glands** are seen on all body sites, and are anatomically independent from the other appendages. Their secretory components are much smaller than those of the apocrine gland, with a smaller lumen (Fig. 2.21). The excretory duct of these glands winds upwards in a spiral pattern through the dermis and the epidermis to the surface.

Fig. 2.18 Growth cycle of scalp hair.

Fig. 2.19 Axillary skin showing large numbers of apocrine glands in the lower third of the section. Apocrine glands are rare in other body sites.

Fig. 2.20 High-power view of secretory cells in apocrine glands showing decapitation pattern of secretion.

Fig. 2.21 Eccrine sweat glands; these will be seen in the deeper dermis in skin from all body sites.

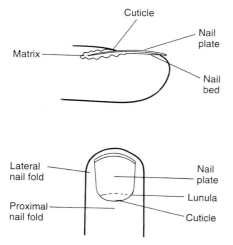

Fig. 2.22 Diagram of the nail and associated structures.

The **nails** are very highly modified skin appendages. The nail itself, or nail plate, grows out from the nail matrix and rests on the underlying nail bed. The pale halo at the proximal end of the nail is called the lunula, and around the edge of this there is a protective rim of cuticle (Fig. 2.22). Nails may become involved in a number of skin diseases, such as psoriasis and fungal infection. The average time for a fingernail to grow out completely from base to outer edge is approximately 6 months, and for toenails the time is 6–18 months or even longer. Thus, therapy of diseased nails requires both time and patience.

Growth point

Apoptosis

The term apoptosis was introduced 20 years ago by Currie, Wylie, and Kerr to describe a type of cell death which at that time was considered unprogrammed. From then until the early 1990s, apoptosis was regarded as a rather abstruse concept with no obvious relevance to most human diseases. In the past few years this has changed dramatically with the realization that apoptosis may be a very important process in tissue modelling, and in removal of potentially malignant cells in the early stages of stepwise progression to malignancy. If the epidermis is examined after exposure to ultraviolet radiation , so called sunburn cells will be seen in the mid epidermis. These are small eosinophilic dead or dying keratinocytes—apoptotic keratinocytes—and the role of apoptosis in ultraviolet induced skin damage and other epidermal disorders is currently under enthusiastic investigation.

Project

Carry out a literature search using the terms apoptosis **and** dermatology/dermatological disease/skin disease. Find out a little about the dermatological diseases which are entered under this heading, and suggest logical reasons for the apoptotic process being necessary here.

What methods are currently available for us to identify the apoptotic cell?

What are the advantages and disadvantages of each of these?

Further reading

Goldsmith, L.A. (ed.) (1983). *Biochemistry and physiology of the skin*, Vol. 1. Oxford University Press, New York.

Rook, A. and Dawber, R. (1982). *Diseases of the hair and scalp*. Blackwell Scientific Publications, Oxford.

Berker, D., Baran, R., and Dawber, R. (1995). *Disease of the nails and their management*. Blackwell Scientific Publications, Oxford.

3

The dermatological history, examination, and investigations frequently used in dermatology

- History-taking
- Examination
- Investigations commonly used in dermatology

History-taking

Most patients with skin disease are seen, and treatment prescribed, in the family doctor's surgery or in a hospital out-patient department. Only a small proportion require admission. It is therefore even more important than in other specialties to ask the patient all the possibly important questions in an orderly and logical framework. Questions forgotten cannot easily be answered until the next visit.

A general outline of useful points to remember in dermatological history-taking include:

1. **How long have any skin lesions been present?** Patients will often only tell you how long they have had the lesions which are currently worrying them and will not begin at the beginning of their problem.
2. **Where did the problem first appear?** As above, patients will often ask you for help only with the patch of psoriasis on their scalp, and will not, unless prompted, tell you about the large plaque on their back. Table 3.1 lists certain common dermatological problems and the likely sites of involvement.
3. **Are there any symptoms?** These are usually itch and/or pain.

   Severe itch is associated with conditions such as:

- scabies
- atopic eczema
- contact dermatitis
- dermatitis herpetiformis.

Key Points

History taking should include; where and when the problem started, symptoms (severe itch, mild itch, pain), medicaments, general medical history, occupation and recreation, travel, family and household contacts, and the patient's own views in the likely cause.

Table 3.1.
Frequent associations between some commoner skin diseases and body sites.

Scalp:	psoriasis, seborrhoeic dermatitis, fungal infections
Face:	atopic dermatitis, acne, rosacea, seborrhoeic dermatitis, lupus erythematosus, and other photosensitive problems
Body flexures:	seborrhoeic dermatitis, psoriasis, fungal infection, candida infection
Feet:	toe webs—fungal infection soles—juvenile plantar dermatosis dorsa—contact dermatitis

Mild itch is associated with many skin conditions including:

- psoriasis
- drug eruptions
- bullous pemphigoid.

Pain is a symptom of vasculitis and pemphigus.

4. **Topical and oral medicament history.** Ask the patient carefully about these. To many elderly patients 'medicines' are not drugs, and the question 'What drugs are you on?' does not always result in an accurate response. Begin by asking about any medicine taken on prescription, then move on to preparations bought over the counter in the chemist or health food shop. An increasing number of patients are using alternative therapy in the form of herbal and homeopathic preparations, and may be reluctant to reveal this in a 'conventional medicine' setting without some coaxing. Ask specifically about sleeping pills, tablets for headaches or other aches and pains, and laxatives.

   In general hospitals, the commonest reason for a request for a dermatologist to see a patient in another ward is because of a suspected adverse drug reaction. Be very sure you have access to a full list of everything given in the past 2–3 weeks, not just the treatment being used on the day you see the patient.

5. **General medical history.** Remember that there are many skin signs which may be the first marker of internal disease (see Chapter 13) and carry out a brief but comprehensive systems enquiry. Diabetes, Crohn's disease, and sarcoidosis can all be first recognized by their dermatological signs provided you know what to look for.

6. **Occupational and recreational history.** Ask about the patient's environment. This may be particularly important in conditions such as contact dermatitis. If the patient is working, an occupational history with brief details of materials handled in a normal working day are useful, but for all patients information about hobbies, recreation, sporting activities, and

Table 3.2.
Possible dermatological occupational and recreational problems

Nursing and hairdressing:	irritant hand dermatitis
Home decorating and repairs:	allergic contact dermatitis from epoxy resin glues
Violinist:	fiddler's neck—acne-like lesions
Sheep farming:	orf from infected animals
Photographic developing:	lichenoid dermatitis from colour developer
Jogging:	Talon noir—small haemorrhages into the thick skin of the heels from ill-fitting shoes

contact with animals may give a clue to the problem. Table 3.2 gives a brief list of possible problems.

Ask also about reaction to sunlight exposure. A number of skin disorders such as lupus erythematosus are initiated or aggravated by sunlight.

7. **Travel**. Ask about holidays, professional travel, and, in the case of those not of UK origin, about visits to or from relatives in their native country. Ask about visits of a relative from overseas, and ask about details of air travel, including refuelling stops. Nowadays many people, including medical students, travel long distances on holiday or to do elective periods of study. A refuelling stop in the Middle East 6 weeks ago may explain the crusted sore on the wrist which is a localized form of leishmaniasis (p. 134).

8. **Family and household contact history**. Many patients with skin disease are confused over infection and genetic transmission. Ask about first-degree relatives as this can be a clue in conditions such as ichthyoses, and also ask about household contacts as these are not always family members. Infections such as scabies may infect both relatives and others with whom the patient is in close contact.

9. **The patient's thoughts on the cause of the problem**. Ask the patient what he or she thinks is wrong and what has caused it. The answer to this question may give you a clue to the diagnosis, and perhaps even more important, may also reveal unexpected theories and worries. Patients may tell you that they believe diet is the cause, and may have tried out unusual and sometimes dangerous dietary changes for themselves or their children. Give the patient time to tell you about this towards the end of the history-taking when he/she is relatively relaxed and you have gained his/her confidence.

These questions should be asked personally in a quiet and unhurried atmosphere where the conversation cannot be overheard by other patients. A 'tick off' questionnaire to fill in while sitting in the waiting room is no substitute for a face-to-face discussion which will, for many patients, be the beginning of therapy.

Remember that almost all patients are embarrassed by skin disease, and many are ashamed of their appearance. Treat them with understanding and sympathy, and they will remember their visits to you with gratitude, even if you cannot yet provide a cure.

Examination

In a few situations—for example, hand warts in children or tinea pedis in athletes—it might just be acceptable to examine only the affected area of the body, but it is a very much better practice to ask all patients attending for the first time to put on a gown and to carry out a total skin examination. If this is done, both related and quite unrelated but potentially serious problems will not be missed and, in the case of the elderly, early curable skin cancers may be identified.

Examine the skin in a good light—daylight if possible—and look carefully at the pattern of involvement of the skin. Many skin diseases have a 'typical' or 'classic' distribution (Fig. 3.1). Draw a sketch in your notes of the affected areas

Key Points

A total skin examination should be carried out to determine the full extent of the problem and possible unrelated conditions.

as this is usually more useful and quicker than detailed notes. Write down the type of skin lesions you see. Dermatologists define primary and secondary lesions, which are outlined in Table 3.3 together with references to where these lesions will be found illustrated in other parts of the book. Is there any sign that the individual lesions have developed on a site of trauma or injury such as a scratch or an operation scar? This is seen in a number of conditions, including psoriasis (p. 44), lichen planus (p. 62), and viral warts (p. 116). This is called the

Fig. 3.1 'Typical' distribution of lesions in common skin disorders.

Atopic Dermatitis (p. 79)

Psoriasis (p. 44)

Acne vulgaris (p. 205)

Light-sensitive eruptions (p. 264)

Seborrhoeic dermatitis (p. 89)

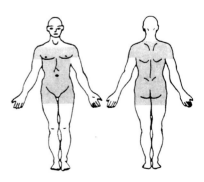

Pityriasis rosea (p. 64)

Table 3.3.
Primary and secondary lesions of the skin

Lesion	Description	Example — where to find it
Primary		
Macule	A flat, circumscribed area of altered skin colour	Vitiligo p. 199, pityriasis versicolor, p. 132 Peutz–Jegher lesions, p. 264
Papule	A small, circumscribed elevation of the skin	Molluscum contagiosum, p. 120
Nodule	A solid, circumscribed elevation whose greater part lies beneath the skin surface	Erythema nodosum, p. 177
Weal	A transient, slightly raised lesion, characteristically with a pale centre and a pink margin	Urticaria, p. 182
Vesicle (blister)	A small (less than 5 mm in diameter), circumscribed, fluid-containing elevation	Dermatitis herpetiformis, p. 235
Bulla (blister)	Similar to a vesicle but larger	Bullous pemphigoid, p. 233
Pustule	A collection of pus	Acne, p. 205
Plaque	A flat-topped palpable lesion	Psoriasis, p. 44
Purpura	Visible collections of free red blood cells	Drug eruption, p. 247
Telangiectasia	Dilated capillaries visible on the skin surface	Topical steroid side-effect, p. 253
Secondary		
Scale	Thickened, loose, readily detached fragments of stratum corneum	Chronic disseminated lupus erythematosus (CDLE), p. 151
Crust	Dried exudate	Impetigo, p. 110
Excoriation	A shallow abrasion often caused by scratching	Atopic eczema, p. 79
Ulcer	An excavation due to loss of tissue including the epidermal surface	p. 174
Scar	A permanent lesion that results from the process of repair by replacement with connective tissue	CDLE, p. 151
Lichenification	Areas of increased epidermal thickness with accentuation of skin	Atopic eczema, p. 79

Koebner phenomenon and is a clue that the mechanisms involved in epidermal healing, possibly growth factors such as transforming growth factor, may be involved in the development of lesions in these diseases.

Remember that very few skin diseases are infectious and do not be afraid of touching the patient's skin. Patients with skin disease often develop a complex that they are 'untouchable' or 'unclean'. Ask the patient about such worries, and about whether or not there are problems with relatives and friends who are concerned about transmission of non-infectious problems such as psoriasis and acne.

Investigations commonly used in dermatology

A number of investigations and ancillary examinations are relatively specific to dermatological practice. It is useful to know what samples are required and what to expect from the laboratory.

Identifying fungal infection

Superficial fungi which cause infections inhabit the outer layer of the skin—the stratum corneum—and skin scales or scrapings should be examined under the microscope. Take a scalpel blade and, with the affected area of skin stretched taut between two fingers, gently scrape the skin with a piece of paper, preferably black, held underneath. Scrape until a reasonable number of silvery scales are on the paper (Fig. 3.2). Try not to cause bleeding by scraping too deeply or too vigorously. This specimen can then be sent at normal temperature through the post if necessary to your local laboratory. Alternatively this specimen can be examined directly, if a microscope is available, on a slide with a drop of 10 per cent potassium hydroxide on it. A network of stick-like fungal hyphae may be seen (Fig. 3.3). Part of the sample should also be sent for culture, which may be positive although no fungi were seen directly, and will allow exact identification of the type of fungus. The result of this test will not be available for 2–3 weeks.

If fungal infection of the hair is suspected, hair brushings, clippings, or scalp scrapings should be treated in the same way. In the case of possible fungal nail infection, take a clipping or scraping from the abnormal area of the nail.

Some fungi (for example *Microsporum canis*) fluoresce brightly under ultraviolet light, and this fact can be used to make an instant diagnosis of scalp ringworm if a Wood's light—a UV source—is available. The fungi will fluoresce bright green.

Fig. 3.2 The technique of taking scrapings for the identification of fungi in the epidermis. A piece of black paper makes it possible to see the scrapings accumulate as the epidermis is gently scraped with a scalpel blade. Do not cause bleeding.

Fig. 3.3 Fungal hyphae. These will be easily seen down the microscope if the skin scrapings are mounted in 10 per cent potassium hydroxide.

Skin biopsy

Many skin conditions require to be biopsied to confirm the clinical diagnosis. This may involve taking a small ellipse of skin with a scalpel (Fig. 3.4) or using a sterile disposable skin biopsy punch with a diameter of 4–8 mm to take a small circle of skin (Fig. 3.5). The punch biopsy technique is extremely quick, and in the case of the smaller samples may not require stitching. However small the biopsy planned, the procedure should be carried out by a clinician with adequate training in an appropriately equipped minor surgery area or biopsy room with excellent lighting and sterile instruments.

Local anaesthetic (1–2 per cent lignocaine preferably without adrenalin) should be infiltrated around the chosen lesion 5 minutes or so before biopsy. Check with a senior colleague about the type of lesion to biopsy, the best site to choose, and the choice of suture material. In general, a fresh lesion is preferred

Fig. 3.4 The use of the scalpel and a skin hook in taking an elliptical skin biopsy. The hook should be inserted at one end of the ellipse and used instead of forceps which will crush the tissue.

Fig. 3.5 The punch biopsy technique. This is quicker than a scalpel biopsy and requires less equipment. A disposable sterile punch 4 mm in diameter is applied with gentle rotating pressure to anaesthetized skin.

(present for less than 24 hours)if the biopsy is to establish the diagnosis, and in the case of, for example, bullous diseases, this is essential. All biopsies will leave a small scar, so try to select a lesion on a site where this will not cause a cosmetic problem, such as the flank. Always try to avoid the shoulders and front of the chest, as the skin on these areas tends to form unsightly keloid scars. Figure 3.6 illustrates the skin tension or Lange's lines. Your biopsy scar should lie along rather than across these lines, as this will give a neater end-result.

What to do with the biopsy specimen

If in doubt, contact the laboratory **before** you begin to biopsy rather than when you are holding the specimen in your hand. Do not guess, as you may be wrong,

Fig. 3.6 Lange's lines. The long axis of a biopsy scar should be oriented along these lines.

and have to explain a day or two later to an unhappy patient that a second biopsy is required.

Most skin biopsies are routinely processed and the specimen should therefore be placed in a fixative such as 10 per cent neutral buffered formalin, clearly labelled, and sent to the laboratory. A number of diseases may also require investigation with immunopathological techniques. These include blistering diseases, connective tissue diseases, and lymphocytic infiltrations in the skin. For these, a small piece of frozen tissue will be required, usually in addition to the fixed sample, and, in the case of infants in whom epidermolysis bullosa is suspected, a sample may also be needed for electron microscopy. Some deep fungal infections may require culture of a biopsy sample to identify the responsible organism.

Confirming the diagnosis of scabies

The female scabies mite or *Acarus* can often be found in the superficial layers of the skin. A good place to look for the mite is the finger webs. A thread-like track may be seen which is the route along which the mite has burrowed into the skin. If the mite can be gently extracted from the skin with a needle, placed on a microscope slide, and the patient invited to examine the cause of his/her itch, you are likely to have a patient who is quite horrified to see the evidence of the cause of his problem and will therefore carry out the prescribed treatment with great attention to detail.

Patch testing to confirm contact dermatitis

Allergic contact dermatitis (p. 96) is a relatively common problem in dermatology clinics. This is caused by a type 4 or lymphocyte mediated immunological reaction, and testing for it is done in vivo, usually using the patients back as the test area. It is important to accurately identify the allergen causing the problem so that the patient can be given instructions about avoidance of materials containing the allergen. If the responsible substance is handled at work, careful reduction of exposure to the material can make all the difference between a patient retaining his job or being forced to seek alternative employment. It is equally important to eliminate substances which the patient feels might be responsible for his problem by negative patch testing results.

Small quantities of a range of potential allergens and also sometimes specially prepared and diluted samples of material the patient has supplied himself are applied to inert metal chambers and large numbers of these—up to 50 is quite feasible—are applied simultaneously to the back (Fig. 3.7). After 48 hours, the patches are removed, and the skin examined for redness and/or swelling both immediately and after another 48 hours (Fig. 3.8). In practice this means the patient being seen three times in one week, on day 1 for application of the patches and on days 3 and 5 for readings.

The exact materials to apply are a specialized area of dermatology, but in Europe the normal practice is to apply 20 substances in the 'European Standard Battery'—the substances found by collaborative research among all European dermatologists to be the most common causes of dermatitis (see p. 99). These are made up in little inert chambers on an adhesive backing. In addition to the

Fig. 3.7 The technique of patch testing. A large number of possible allergens have been applied to the back. Note the use of dye as a site marker.

Fig. 3.8 A positive patch test showing erythema at 96 hours after application of the patches.

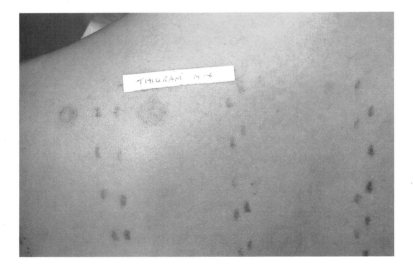

Standard European Battery, specialist sets of materials are available for certain body sites (e.g. footwear) or occupations (hairdressers, photographers).

In North America, a slightly different set of allergens is used and monitored by the North American Contact Dermatitis Group.

'Allergy tests'

Many patients or parents of children with atopic dermatitis and urticaria in particular request allergy tests in the belief that it is possible to identify the allergen(s) involved in these conditions and that, if these are then avoided, a cure will result. Unfortunately, this is not always feasible. Type 1 allergy tests or prick tests may identify clinically relevant allergens in respiratory atopy, but the patient with cutaneous problems will usually react on prick testing to many allergens, for example, house dust mite, pollens, cat and dog hair, and protein foodstuffs. The relevance of these reactions to the patient's dermatological problems is often doubtful and, for this reason, few dermatology departments will routinely carry out such tests.

The quantitation of circulating serum IgE, measuring both total and specific IgE levels to inhaled and ingested allergens, using the radio allergo sorbent or RAST test is a little more relevant, but again it may not be of practical value in that vigorous avoidance of all the allergens giving rise to a positive RAST may not improve the condition, and conversely continued exposure to, for example, dog hair to which a positive RAST result has been obtained may cause no problems. Careful clinical observation on the part of both doctor and patient or parent is more likely to produce clinically relevant information.

Photography

In dermatological records, one well-taken clinical photograph is frequently worth several paragraphs, and photographs are usually required if you are planning to present the case at a grand round, clinical meeting, or to write a case report for a journal.

Choose appropriate lighting and make sure there are no flowery curtains in the background or disconcerting clothing in the foreground. Be sure that the picture illustrates both the site and the details of the problem, and use a centimetre scale laid on the skin for close-up views. If you have access to a medical illustration department, be present when the photograph is being taken to show the photographer exactly what is required, and always ask the patient's permission. In many centres nowadays, this permission is given in writing, and this certainly should be done if you are planning to use the photograph in a publication.

Project

Find out where the pathology and mycology samples from the patients you see are processed and reported. If possible, follow some of these samples from the time they are taken from the patient to the writing of the report in the laboratory.

What have you learned about:

1. how to take a useful sample;

2. the details needed on the request form;

3. how to make contact if a report received is difficult to interpret?

Further reading

Myerscough, P.R. (1989). *Talking with patients*. Oxford University Press, Oxford.

Zachary, C.B. (1991). *Basic cutaneous surgery*. Churchill Livingstone, New York.

Robinson, J. (1986). *Fundamentals of skin biopsy*. Chicago Year Book Publications.

Lawrence, C.M. and Cox, N.H. (1993). *Physical signs in dermatology*. Wolfe London.

4

Psoriasis, other papulosquamous diseases, and disorders of keratinization

- Psoriasis

- Lichen planus

- Pityriasis rosea

- Pityriasis rubra pilaris

- Darier's disease

- The ichthyoses: autosomal dominant ichthyosis vulgaris X-linked recessive ichthyosis bullous ichthyosiform erythroederma

Problem cases

Read these case presentations, work your way through the information in this chapter, talk if possible to patients with similar problems, carry out an appropriate literature search if you have the facilities, and only then read the suggested management plans on page 76.

Case 4.1

A 36-year-old, newly married accountant consults you about the management of her persistent widespread plaque psoriasis. She first developed psoriatic lesions when she was 14, and there is a strong family history. Although she attended the local specialist as a teenager 20 years ago, she found the rather messy tar preparations then prescribed unacceptable, and has not sought medical help for the last 15 years. She uses a little emollient to reduce scaling and wears clothing which covers her knees and elbows, which are particularly troublesome. She wants to know if there are any new advances in psoriasis treatment which would help her, and in passing mentions that she hopes to start a family within the next year.

What are the treatment options which might be appropriate in this case?

Case 4.2

A 73-year-old widower who lives alone has hypertension, chronic obstructive airways disease, and extensive widespread psoriasis which is at times erythrodermic. In the past, a ten day admission to the local hospital once or twice annually has kept his skin at least partly under control, but local bed reductions mean that this is no longer available. He finds applying topical therapy to his body regularly very difficult both because of his breathlessness and arthritis in his hands.

What treatment regimes might be appropriate here? He is determined to continue to live in his own home.

Case 4.3

A 58-year-old woman comes to you with itchy papules on one wrist. They have been present for about 6 weeks. She thinks they may be insect bites. Her only medication is a diuretic which she has been on for 3 years for mild hypertension.

What conditions would you consider in the differential diagnosis, and how would you establish a diagnosis?

Case 4.4

A 21-year-old male is brought to you by his girl friend. They have just returned from a sunny holiday on which he was badly sunburned. His back is covered with infected, crusted lesions and he feels generally unwell.

What conditions might this history suggest, and how would you arrive at a diagnosis?

Case 4.5

A 24-year-old male is referred by a colleague for your advice. The young man has had psoriasis since infancy, and has never responded well to topical tar or dithranol preparations. In the past 2 years, he has had systemic treatment with PUVA and retinoids, again with no benefit. Your colleague wants to know if you would consider oral methotrexate justified, despite the patients age.

How would you reply?

Key Points

Psoriasis affects at least 1–3 per cent of Caucasians.

Psoriasis

Psoriasis is one of the commonest of all skin diseases. All doctors need to be familiar with the many different types of clinical presentation, and to know the currently available range of treatments with their advantages and disadvantages.

Definition

A chronic relapsing and remitting scaling skin disease which may appear at any age and affect any part of the skin surface.

Prevalence

Among Caucasians, the prevalence of psoriasis is about 1–3 per cent. This is probably a significant underestimate, first, because patients with mild psoriasis may not seek medical help, and, second, because incidence figures are often derived from hospital records so that those treated solely by family doctors or choosing to live with their disease will be excluded.

The sexes are affected equally and there appear to be two subgroups, one with onset most commonly in the second decade, and one with onset in the fourth and fifth decades. Some workers subdivide psoriasis on the basis of age of onset into psoriasis type 1 and type 2. Type 1 psoriasis patients, with the earlier age of onset, have a stronger family history, and a higher frequency of HLA CW6 and B13 antigens (see below).

Aetiology

It is clear that there are both inherited and environmental factors which influence the development of psoriasis. Although a very wide range of bio-chemical and pathological abnormalities have been reported in psoriatic skin, the exact cause of psoriasis is not yet known. Table 4.1 lists some of the reported abnormalities in the skin of psoriatic patients. A major problem, however, is the need to establish whether or not these observed abnormalities are primary or secondary. In studies of psoriasis it is common to use for comparison two pieces

Table 4.1.

Abnormalities found in psoriatic skin with possible explanations

Abnormalities	Comment
Accelerated transit time of keratinocytes through the epidermis	The most consistent observation in psoriatic skin
Increased mitotic activity	Not only the basal layer
Increased rate of DNA synthesis	keratinocytes, but also cells two or three layer above
Increased levels of phospholipase A_2 activity	Availability of fee arachidonic acid. High levels LTB_4 may explain pustules in psoriatic lesions
Elevated levels of polyamine synthesis	May well be secondary to rapid cell proliferation
Increased levels of plasminogen activator	May explain Koebner phenomenon
Presence of keratins 6 and 16 in epidermis	Probably secondary to accelerated transit time
Increased cGMP levels leading to high ratio cGMP/cAMP	
High levels of calcium binding protein calmodulin	Both cyclosporin and dithranol are calmodulin antagonists

of control skin—absolutely normal control tissue from a non-psoriatic patient and also clinically normal skin from a patient with psoriasis. If the clinically normal psoriatic skin also shows the abnormality, it is likely to be a primary rather than a secondary abnormality. However, the fact that this abnormality is seen in skin which is not clinically abnormal indicates that an additional factor or factors are needed for development of the psoriatic lesion.

Genetics of psoriasis

Genetic factors play a role in the pathogenesis of psoriasis and approximately one-third of patients have a positive family history. Twin studies suggest that the pattern of inheritance is multifactorial and that environmental factors may be required for clinical expression of latent disease. Recent studies on the human leucocyte antigen (HLA) system have shown an association, in Caucasians, between psoriasis and both HLA–CW6 and HLA–DR7. Patients with pustular psoriasis have a higher than normal incidence of the HLA–B27 antigen. A recent study of 65 psoriasis patients in 8 families has suggested that one of the genes coding for increased susceptibility to psoriasis may be located on the long arm of chromosome 17.

Transforming growth factor alpha

Several studies have now confirmed that there is abnormal expression of transforming growth factor alpha in psoriatic epidermis, and that this reverts to normal during treatments of various types. At present, there is a lot of interest in epidermal abnormalities in transgenic mouse models where the human TGF alpha gene has been introduced, and also in the relationship between abnormalities of TGF alpha expression and abnormalities of integrin expression, as these are also seen in psoriasis.

Calcium metabolism and psoriasis

Abnormalities of calcium metabolism may play a part in psoriasis. Calmodulin is a calcium binding protein which may be elevated in the serum of some patients with active psoriasis, and may fall with treatment. Topical calcipotriol (p. 58) is a newer topical therapy for psoriasis, and the suggested mode of action is that it promotes normal differentiation in the psoriatic epidermis.

Epidermal keratinocyte proliferation in psoriasis

There is no doubt that psoriatic plaques have an increased epidermal cell proliferation rate. Radiolabelling techniques have been used to measure the transit time of epidermal cells maturing in their transit through the skin. In normal skin this is about 50–75 days, whereas in psoriatic skin it is only 8–10 days. With similar techniques, it has been shown that, while the germinative component of normal human epidermis is confined to the basal layer, in psoriatic skin it comprises the lower three layers of epidermal cells. It seems, therefore, that the rapid turnover of psoriatic cells is due not only to an increase in the number of actively dividing cells, but also to an acceleration in their rate of reproduction. As has been explained in Chapter 2, p. 15 the two pairs of keratins found in the basal cells of normal epidermis are keratins 5 and 14, while keratins 1 and 10 predominate in the suprabasal layers. In psoriasis there is a persistence above the basal layer of keratins 5 and 14, and in addition keratins 6 and 16 are seen. These are keratins associated with rapid cell division and tissue repair.

Immunological aspects of psoriasis

Immunological aspects of psoriasis have also stimulated aetiological theories based on the concept that psoriatic keratinocytes have an abnormal surface antigen which, when exposed to the immune system, triggers off an immune response. Antibodies against abnormal keratin are produced, and, when immune complexes are formed, an inflammatory reaction results. The fact that the immunosuppressive drug cyclosporin is an effective method of controlling psoriasis (see below) is also contributory evidence that an immune response may play a part in the development of the psoriatic lesion.

The Koebner phenomenon

It is possible, partly, to explain the Koebner or isomorphic phenomenon in immunological terms. The Koebner phenomenon describes the tendency for psoriatic lesions to develop at sites of skin trauma, such as mechanical friction, sunburn, or lesions of childhood illnesses such as chickenpox. Possibly, the abnormal or unstable keratinocyte surface antigens or the abnormal keratin formed in those who are genetically predisposed are exposed, by trauma, to the immune system which then reacts, triggering a hyperproliferative response in the epidermis.

Systemic drugs and psoriasis

Psoriasis may be both aggravated and precipitated for the first time by some systemic drugs. These include lithium, and some antihypertensive agents including beta blockers. Patients with psoriasis planning a tropical holiday must be aware that the antimalarial chloroquine may cause their psoriasis to deteriorate. Alternatives, such paludrine and mefloquine, do not cause this problem.

Infection and psoriasis

Streptococcal infection, usually in the form of a sore throat, is a well recognized precipitating event in patients with guttate psoriasis. It has been suggested that this may be due to the presence of superantigens and that there are shared antigens between the wall of the streptococcus and the keratinocyte.

Ultraviolet radiation and psoriasis

The majority of patients with psoriasis find that their lesions improve on exposure to natural sunlight, but about 15 per cent find that UV exposure aggravates pre-existing lesions and may stimulate the development of new lesions. To date no clear biochemical or immunological explanation has been proposed for these two subsets of psoriasis patients with opposing responses to UV.

Stress, smoking, and alcohol

In common with many skin conditions, psoriasis may develop for the first time during periods of stress, or stress may aggravate pre-existing lesions. The reason for this is not yet understood. Both smoking and a high alcohol intake are associated with psoriasis, but to what extent this is because of the disease rather than a cause of it in the first place is debated.

Pathology

The difference between normal epidermis and papillary dermis and that seen in active psoriatic lesions is shown diagrammatically in Fig. 4.1. The stratum corneum in psoriasis contains nuclei and is therefore parakeratotic. There is no granular layer, and the prickle cell layer is expanded with bulbous, downward projections. Mitotic figures may be seen in suprabasal keratinocytes. In the papillary dermis, large dilated thin-walled blood vessels will be seen and above these vessels

Fig. 4.1 Psoriatic and normal skin compared.

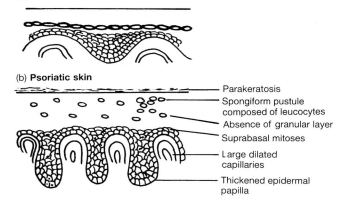

(a) **Normal skin**

(b) **Psoriatic skin**

— Parakeratosis
— Spongiform pustule composed of leucocytes
— Absence of granular layer
— Suprabasal mitoses
— Large dilated capillaries
— Thickened epidermal papilla

Fig. 4.2 Classic untreated lesions of psoriasis vulgaris. These lesions are commonly seen on the knees, elbows, and sacrum, and present as plaques topped by white or silvery scales.

Fig. 4.3 Psoriasis of the elbows showing striking erythema and scaling.

the epidermis is often relatively thin. In both the dermis and epidermis there may be an infiltrate of leucocytes, and these may clump together in the stratum corneum to form so-called **Munro microabscesses or spongiform pustules.**

Clinical features

Clinically recognized types of psoriasis include:

- **classic plaque psoriasis**
- **guttate**
- **seborrhoeic, flexural napkin, or inversus**
- **erythrodermic**
- **pustular**—generalized (von Zumbusch) or localized on the trunk and limbs or plamoplantar.

Plaque psoriasis

Classically, psoriasis vulgaris presents as erythematous, scaly plaques, involving most commonly the extensor aspects of the knees (Fig. 4.2), and elbows (Fig. 4.3), and the scalp (Fig. 4.4). Other common sites are the hands and the sacral area. The total area affected ranges from a few tiny plaques to almost all the body surface (Figs 4.5, 4.6, and 4.7). Untreated, the individual lesions are elevated, palpable, and topped by greyish-white or micaceous scale. Rubbing them after gently removing the scale reveals pin-point bleeding from the dilated, superficial capillaries (Auspitz' sign). These dilated capillaries in the dermis can be seen on histological examination of a psoriatic plaque.

Guttate psoriasis

Guttate or 'raindrop' psoriasis is commoner in children than in adults, and presents as multiple small psoriatic lesions mainly on the trunk. This pattern is frequently preceded by a streptococcal throat infection (Fig. 4.8). It is quite

Fig. 4.4 Psoriasis of the scalp. This can be difficult to treat and can cause some hair thinning.

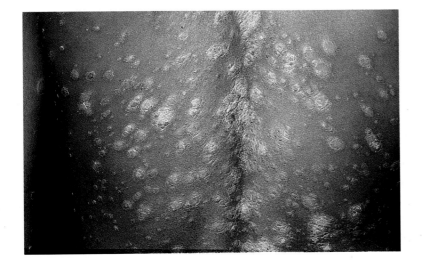

Fig. 4.5 Psoriatic plaques on the back of an individual with coloured skin.

common for a young patient to have only one episode of guttate psoriasis and thereafter no further problems.

Seborrhoeic psoriasis

Seborrhoeic psoriasis or **psoriasis inversus** are descriptive terms applicable when classical psoriatic lesions on the scalp are associated with less typical erythematous, finely scaling lesions in the body folds, especially the groins, axillae, and inframammary regions. Diagnosis may be difficult on both clinical and histological grounds, as the erythema and scaling can be very similar to that seen in seborrhoeic dermatitis. Similarly, napkin psoriasis in infants tends to involve the creases in the groin and is seen as red areas with associated fine scaling rather than the classic more clearly demarcated psoriatic plaque. Psoriasis involving the

Fig. 4.6 Erythematus psoriatic plaques on a Caucasian back.

Fig. 4.7 Extensive psoriatic plaques developing on the trunk after chicken pox.

Fig. 4.8 Extensive guttate psoriasis.

Fig. 4.9 Erythrodermic psoriasis involving mainly the lower part of the abdominal skin.

body flexures can be difficult to treat as it is easily irritated by topical tars and dithranol which are very effective in other sites.

Erythrodermic psoriasis

Erythrodermic psoriasis presents as an extensive erythema of the entire body surface with, at times, very few classical scaling psoriatic lesions (Fig. 4.9). Grossly increased blood flow through the skin may lead to loss of thermo-regulation and to high output cardiac failure.

Pustular psoriasis

Pustular psoriasis refers to varieties of psoriasis in which sterile pustules are an obvious clinical feature. When present they tend to occur at the advancing edge of psoriatic lesions (Fig. 4.10). They may also be seen in erythrodermic psoriasis and the combination of extensive erythroderma and sterile pustules is termed the **von Zumbusch** type of pustular psoriasis, a serious and, at times, life-threatening variety due to associated fluid and electrolyte imbalance and high output cardiac decompensation. Pustular psoriasis may also be seen as a non-life-threatening, but extremely chronic variant, on the palms and soles. These lesions respond poorly to currently available therapy (Fig. 4.11).

Although psoriasis has been said to be asymptomatic, many patients with ac-tively developing lesions complain of pruritus. Scratching may cause fresh lesions due to the Koebner phenomenon. After the first attack of psoriasis, relapses and remissions are frequent. A few fortunate individuals, after a single episode of guttate psoriasis, enter an almost complete and prolonged remission. More com-monly, however, mild involvement of the scalp, knees, and elbows persists with, at varying intervals, episodes of more widespread involvement. Some psoriatics find their lesions improve over the years, whilst in others the process becomes more widespread and troublesome. Childhood psoriasis, although less common than in adults, tends to be both persistent and difficult to treat.

Fig. 4.10 Close-up of an expanding plaque of pustular psoriasis showing classic pustulation at the edge of the lesion.

Fig. 4.11 Pustular psoriasis of the soles. The pustules are sterile.

Scalp involvement

Psoriasis of the scalp is seen as thick, obvious scaling and redness, often most obvious at the hairline and behind the ears. Some patients with long-standing scalp psoriasis develop a degree of hair thinning, but it is not clear whether this is due to the psoriatic process *per se* or to treatment.

Nail involvement

A proportion of patients with long-standing psoriasis develop nail changes, including small pits on the nail plate and separation of part of the nail from the nail bed (onycholysis) with subungual hyperkeratosis. Discoloration of the nail resembling grease spots is also seen (Figs 4.12, 4.13, and 4.14).

Psoriatic arthropathy

This is a distinctive seronegative arthropathy usually seen in patients with established cutaneous lesions of psoriasis. The sacro-iliac and distal interphalangeal joints are most commonly involved, but any joint may be affected by this mutilating variety of arthropathy. A higher incidence of arthropathy is seen in those with psoriatic nail changes. Occasionally, psoriatic arthropathy is diagnosed in the absence of overt skin lesions, but this is rare and other causes of arthropathy must first be carefully excluded.

Fig. 4.12 Typical psoriatic nail changes. Note the separation of the distal part of the nail from the underlying nail plate (oncholysis) and the pitting of the nail.

Fig. 4.13 Severe psoriasis of the hands with associated nail involvement.

Fig. 4.14 Severe destructive psoriasis of the finger nails.

Differential diagnosis

This includes Reiter's disease, lichen planus, seborrhoeic dermatitis, pityriasis rosea, and pityriasis rubra pilaris. Reiter's disease (p. 141) can usually be excluded in the absence of genitourinary, rheumatological, or gastrointestinal complaints. The histological features are diagnostic in lichenoid reactions including lichen planus (p. 62) so if in doubt a biopsy is justified. The histology of seborrhoeic dermatitis will usually, but not always, differentiate between this and seborrhoeic psoriasis. Biopsy and histological examination will differentiate pityriasis rosea and pityriasis rubra pilaris from psoriasis.

Be cautious about diagnosing an isolated plaque on the trunk of an elderly patient as psoriasis. Bowen's disease (p. 289) may look very similar. Once again, a biopsy will establish the correct diagnosis.

Investigations

Patients presenting with classic plaque psoriasis can easily be diagnosed on clinical grounds, and a biopsy is not indicated unless there is clinical doubt. Occasionally, particularly when the presenting feature is a scaling lesion of the palm, taking scrapings for mycological examination to exclude a fungal infection is wise. Also in any patient with psoriasis and joint pain, radiological examination and taking blood samples for rheumatoid factor and antinuclear antibody assessment is indicated.

Treatment

In considering appropriate treatment for a patient with psoriasis it is important to consider:

- the patient's age and general health, including, if female, plans for pregnancy;

- the type of psoriasis;

- the body surface area involved and the areas worst affected

- the previous treatments used and their success or failure

- what the patient hopes for and needs to achieve for his/ her life-style.

This last point is important and should be discussed with the patient at his/her first visit. An elderly patient with knee and elbow problems may only wish to spend time applying topical therapy for 2 or 3 weeks before an annual holiday, whereas a 20-year-old ballet dancer may need to keep her skin completely clear in order to pursue her career.

It is important at the time of the first consultation to explain to the patient the usually chronic nature of psoriasis and the fact that currently available treatments *control* rather than cure the disease. The need for the patient's own active involvement, and possibly also that of a relative, in topical treatment should be explained. Recently there have been attempts to quantitate the degree of dermatological disability caused by a number of skin conditions, and the psoriasis disability index is a well developed questionnaire on such items as time lost from work, interpersonal relations, and other problems which were found on a much more detailed questionnaire to be the most common problems affecting the majority of psoriasis patients. This questionnaire administered before and after treatment can give some guide to the patients view of the value of his treatment.

Many patients have unspoken fears that their psoriasis is infectious, or a form of cancer, or even both of these. The difference between an inherited susceptibility, which is present in psoriasis, and truly contagious infection such as impetigo may require explanation and the truly non-malignant and even non-premalignant nature of psoriasis should be emphasized.

Clear, useful patient information sheets are available on psoriasis. These are helpful and will reinforce the instructions given at the original consultation as much of this may be quickly forgotten.

Once the nature of the disease is fully understood, many patients with mild psoriasis may prefer to leave small plaques on knees and elbows untreated. There

Key Points

Appropriate treatment for psoriasis depends on the patient's situation, type and extent of psoriasis, previous treatment and level of control desired.

is no evidence that this will cause extension of psoriasis and it is an entirely acceptable option. A mild emollient, such as emulsifying ointment BP or white soft paraffin, will minimize scaling.

The majority of patients with psoriasis, however, will require a more active treatment programme. Methods of managing psoriasis have advanced considerably in the past few years, and the range of available topical and systemic therapies are itemized in Table 4.2 and examples of their use in Table 4.3.

The great majority of patients will use topical therapy in their own homes, and it is well worthwhile arranging a demonstration by a trained dermatological nurse of exactly how to use the creams and ointments prescribed, either in the surgery, office, outpatient clinic, or in an outpatient treatment centre. A high proportion of apparent non-responses to appropriate antipsoriatic therapy are due to patients not understanding how to apply their treatment, how thick a layer to apply, how to use covering bandages and dressings, and how to prevent irritation of surrounding normal skin. Many dermatology departments now have out-patient treatment centres where patients with more severe or extensive psoriasis can attend for out-patient phototherapy and help with dressings, and only those with very extensive, or erythrodermic, or pustular psoriasis will require inpatient care. This does put an additional burden of care of psoriasis patients on community services, and the use of dermatology community liaison nurses needs to be extended.

Topical therapy

This is the main form of treatment for the great majority of psoriasis patients. Appropriate preparations include:

- emollients
- tar preparations
- dithranol preparations
- calciptriol
- salicylic acid preparations
- topical steroids.

Emollients

Emollients are of great value in psoriasis in minimizing scaling, and preventing the development of cracks and hacks. Patients should be given a pack of small samples of several emollients to try and choose the most effective for their skin. Usually a lighter preparation is preferred for the trunk and limbs, and a heavier one for the hands and feet. This will reduce scaling but will not affect erythema or the basic psoriatic process.

Tar preparations

These have been used to treat psoriasis for over 100 years and appear to have antimitotic activity. They are available as creams, pastes, and ointments, and need to be covered with stockinet dressings. Evidence based dermatology and

Table 4.2.

Topical and systemic preparations of value in the management of psoriasis

	Preparation	Advantages	Disadvantages
Topical therapy	Dithranol-based	Long term safety data reassuring	Some staining and irritation common. Difficult for out-patient use
	Tar	Long term safety data reassuring	Messy and cosmetically relatively unacceptable. Recent concern about carcinogenicity
	Salicylic acid	Useful particularly for scalps, and hyperkeratotic palms and soles	Danger of salicylicism if high concentrations used on large areas of the body
	Topical steroids	Clean and cosmetically acceptable	Only moderate potency acceptable. Risk of topical side effects with more potent preparations
	Calcipotriol	Cosmetically acceptable	Very useful in primary care but of value only in mild to moderate psoriasis. Tends to improve but not completely clear lesions
	Ultraviolet light UVB-natural sunlight wavelengths	Cosmetically acceptable	Unknown future risk of malignancy. Improvement in psoriatic lesions tends to be associated with some erythema.
Systemic therapy	Photochemotherapy (Psoralens + UVA = PUVA)	Cosmetically acceptable	Definite risk of malignancy (squamous cell carcinoma) in patients who have had more than 500 treatments
	Cytotoxic drugs (methotrexate, azathioprine, hydroxyurea)	Rapidly effective	Teratogenicity. Liver, marrow and renal toxicity
	Retinoid group of drugs Acetretin (Neotigason)	Effective in 50% of chronic plaque psoriasis. Very effective in 80% of pustular psoriasis of palms and soles	Teratogenicity. Raised serum lipids. Cheilitis. Bony changes
	Cyclosporin (Neoral)	Effective	Rapid rebound on stopping treatment. Risk of permanent renal damage.

Table 4.3.

Examples of treatment for psoriasis of different types in different age ranges

Patient	Types of Psoriasis	Special considerations	Treatment	Comments
Boy aged 10	Guttate psoriasis	Usually self-healing type of psoriasis	0.1% dithranol in cream base or simple white soft paraffin	Check for recurrent sore throats and enlarged tonsils
Married woman aged 28	Chronic plaque	Wishes to add to family	Primary care trial of topical calcipotriol ointment. If ineffective, short contact dithranol up to 2% 30 minutes daily	No currently available systemic treatment is appropriate for women who wish to become pregnant
Male aged 40	Severe pustular lesions	Hand lesions causing concern over losing job	Trial of topical dithranol. If not successful try topical steroids if these fail, consider for systemic Acetretin therapy	
Female aged 56	Widespread plaques	Four recent hospital admissions. Post-menopausal. Relatively dithranol-resistant	Consider for PUVA therapy	Appropriate only if patient lives reasonably close to PUVA centre. It is essential to keep an accurate record of the number of UVA exposures and the total dose of UVA
Male aged 72	Erythrodermic psoriasis	Severe chronic obstructive airway diseases makes home use of topical preparations very difficult	Consider methotrexate	Possible hepatic toxicity may be outweighed by improved quality of life.

recent comparative clinical trials suggest that the maximum benefit from topical tar will be achieved by concentrations no higher than 5 per cent and that there is no logical reason to use higher concentrations which are messy, and stain both clothing and bedding. A few patients develop a sterile folliculitis when tar is applied to hair-bearing areas. This is self-limiting.

The traditional Goeckermann regime includes the use of both tar and ultraviolet light (UVB), and there is some evidence to suggest that the combination of UVB and tar will clear psoriatic plaques more quickly than either alone.

There are a large number of cleaner proprietary tar preparations available. These are slightly less effective than crude coal tar preparations, but for out-patient use this is more than compensated for by their cosmetic acceptability. These include 5 per cent tar and 2 per cent allantoin in a 'vanishing cream' base (Alphosyl), Clinitar, Pragmatar; 10 per cent tar in a water miscible base (Carbodome), and Zetar (USA).

Tar is a recognized carcinogen and from time to time public concern is expressed about its safety in psoriasis, and the possibility raised that short-term advantage in the clearance of psoriatic plaques might be at the expense of increased risk of either cutaneous or systemic malignancy. Long-term studies of patients with psoriasis from many parts of the world, show no evidence that tar treatment adds to cancer risk. In contrast, the excess cigarette smoking, so common in many patients with psoriasis, is a real carcinogenic hazard.

Dithranol (anthralin)

Preparations containing dithranol act in psoriasis by inhibiting mitosis and thus slowing down the excessive rate of keratinocyte division in psoriasis. They are widely used and are useful for most types of psoriasis. The concentration of dithranol used may vary from 0.1 to 3 per cent or higher in an appropriate base. This is commonly Lassar's paste (zinc paste with 15 per cent salicylic acid added). Traditionally, this paste has been applied to psoriatic plaques night and morning under a stockinet gauze dressing after protecting the surrounding normal skin with white soft paraffin, a very important point in patient education, as normal non-psoriatic skin is easily irritated by dithranol. The Ingram regime combines topical dithranol applications with tar baths and ultraviolet light therapy (UVB). This treatment is safe and effective, with psoriatic plaques clearing in 2–3 weeks. As the psoriatic lesions clear, the skin may temporarily become stained a grey-brown colour. This staining wears off 7–10 days after stopping treatment.

Ready prepared dithranol preparations in the UK include a range of concentrations of dithranol in Dithrolan and Dithrocream, and also Psoradrate, which contains urea. In the USA an equivalent proprietary preparation is Drithocream.

Dithranol—short contact treatment

A popular, patient-acceptable, and effective method of applying dithranol is by the 'short contact' technique which is based on the observation that dithranol applied to plaques of psoriasis remains on the psoriatic epidermis in small quantities after washing.

In the short contact regime, the patient applies the appropriate concentration of dithranol (usually between 0.25 and 1 per cent) to his skin for 10–30 minutes daily and after this time bathes or showers to remove all visible dithranol. This can be done in the early morning or late evening and is a very convenient approach, avoiding the need for dressings or staining of clothing. Comparative studies have shown that this approach will result in a slightly longer time taken to clear the lesions than traditional 24-hour contact with bandaging, but the greater convenience of short contact therapy compensates for this for most patients.

Calciptriol or calcipotriene (Dovonex)

Calciptriol is a vitamin D analogue synthesized for topical use. It has very little effect in mobilizing the body's calcium stores, and therefore hypercalcaemia has only been observed to date in patients who have used very large quantities for long periods of time. It is thought to act by promoting normal epidermal differentiation. Patients using calciptriol notice a rapid reduction in scaling of their psoriatic plaques, and a slower reduction in underlying erythema which does not always clear completely. It has the advantage of being clean and odour free and is therefore justifiably popular for out-patient use. The current recommendation is that no more than 100 g weekly should be used to avoid any risk of hypercalcaemia. Both a cream and a scalp application are currently available.

Salicylic acid-containing preparations

These are most commonly used on the scalp, and on very thick hyperkeratotic areas on the palms and soles. Salicylic acid is a keratolytic and is used on the scalp in concentrations of 10–20 per cent in aqueous cream or emulsifying ointment; and in lower concentrations for the palms and soles. If it is used over large body areas in high concentrations absorption could lead to salicylism.

Topical steroids

Sensibly used, topical steroids are useful in the management of psoriasis in certain body sites. They should never, however, be the mainstay of treatment of chronic plaque psoriasis. Although the plaques will initially respond, in time many patients will develop 'unstable' or erythrodermic psoriasis. Other problems of inappropriate long-term steroid use are described on p. 253.

Moderate potency topical steroids are, however, useful for the management of flexural psoriasis provided the duration of use is carefully controlled. Pustular psoriasis of the palms and soles may respond to stronger topical steroids—for example beclomethasone dipropionate (Propaderm) or fluocinolone acetonide (Synalar)—and here also the quantity of steroid used and the duration of treatment should be carefully monitored.

Combinations of topical steroids and other antipsoriatic preparations described above can be useful. The combination of a topical steroid and salicylic acid (Diprosalic) is useful as a lotion for stubborn scalp psoriasis.

Other steroid-containing gels and lotions (for example Betnovate scalp application, Synalar gel) are clean and easy to use, but quantities prescribed should be reviewed regularly and, in the case of chronic persistent lesions, alternatives such as Cocois (12 per cent coal tar solution, 2 per cent salicylic acid, 4 per cent precipitated sulphur in coconut oil and wax) considered.

Ultraviolet light (UVB)

The action of both tar and dithranol is enhanced by exposure to ultraviolet light in the UVB range (280–315 nm). These are the predominant wavelengths found in natural sunlight, and are usually administered in carefully measured doses from appropriate light sources in the Goeckermann regime with tar, or the Ingram regime with dithranol. Newer developments suggest that so called narrow band UVB, using tubes emitting ultraviolet radiation only in the 310–312 nm range, is even more effective in rapidly clearing psoriatic plaques.

Shampoos

While it is traditional to prescribe tar-based and salicylic acid containing shampoos for mild psoriasis, there is little proof of their efficacy by comparison with regular use of a standard shampoo. Some patients find them soothing, but to be effective they must be left in contact with the scalp for several minutes. In many countries tar containing shampoos are only available on prescription because of the theoretical risk of carcinogenesis. At present in the UK, they are available without prescription, although there have been reports of tar breakdown products in the peripheral blood after applications of only 5 minutes.

Systemic therapy

- PUVA photochemotherapy

- Oral retinoids

- Methotrexate

- Cyclosporin

- Hydroxyurea

- Systemic steroids

While topical therapy properly applied will control the great majority of psoriatic lesions, a small proportion of patients will require more potent systemic therapy. The choices here lie between photochemotherapy (PUVA), the retinoid group of drugs (currently only available in the UK on hospital prescription), cytotoxic drugs (including methotrexate and hydroxyurea), and the immunosuppressive cyclosporin. These treatments should not be considered until a very adequate trial of topical treatment has failed. None are safe for women in the child-bearing years without adequate (usually oral) contraception. Systemic steroids should only very rarely be used to control psoriasis. Although initially effective, the dosage needed to maintain control rises steadily, and patients end up suffering more from the side-effects of systemic steroid therapy than they ever would from psoriasis.

Fig. 4.15 A typical photochemotherapy (PUVA) cabinet.

Photochemotherapy (PUVA)

This treatment involves the use of an oral photosensitizing agent, a psoralen, and subsequent total body exposure 2 hours later to ultraviolet light in the UVA range (320–365 nm; psoralen + UVA = PUVA) in a specially designed cabinet (Fig. 4.15). This form of therapy should only be used for clearing psoriasis—induction therapy. Growing evidence of the increased risk of non-melanoma skin cancer associated with high dose long-term PUVA means that maintenance PUVA therapy is not now recommended, and that an upper lifetime limit of 1000 J/m^2 prescribed UVA is recommended. The combination of both oral retinoids and PUVA—RePUVA—is for some patients an effective method of psoriasis control which allows lower doses of both UV and retinoids to be given. The normal pattern is to start oral retinoid treatment 10–14 days before introducing PUVA.

Psoralen is deposited in the lens of the eye and PUVA-treated patients must therefore wear dark glasses during treatment and for 24 hours thereafter.

Retinoids

Retinoids are synthetic vitamin A-like derivatives. The retinoid currently commercially available and most effective for disorders of keratinization is acetretin (Neotigason, Neotegason). The exact mode of action is not understood but it is well recognized that vitamin A is necessary for normal keratinization. The usual starting dose is 25–30 mg orally daily for 2–4 weeks. Some heavier patients will require a slightly higher dose. Neotigason can be used relatively long term to control psoriasis provided patients are carefully monitored. Minor side-effects include drying of the lips and nasal mucosa and are easily dealt with by the liberal use of emollients. Retinoids may be associated with elevation of serum cholesterol and triglycerides, and assessment of fasting lipids pre-treatment and thereafter at 3–6 month intervals is therefore wise. The most important point is that retinoids are teratogenic, and that young female patients must use a totally reliable form of contraception, both during retinoid therapy and for 2 years after cessation of therapy, as retinoids can be stored for long periods in the body fat. The implication of this is that Neotigason is not appropriate psoriasis therapy for a younger female who has not yet completed her family.

As indicated under PUVA, the combination of retinoid and PUVA can be effective and reduce total dose requirements of either preparation.

Methotrexate

Methotrexate is a very useful cytotoxic drug for control of severe psoriasis. Control can usually be obtained with relatively small doses given at weekly intervals. Its particular advantage is its speed of action, as improvement of psoriasis may be seen within 48 hours of administration of methotrexate.

Methotrexate can be given orally, intramuscularly, or intravenously. The usual dose required varies from 5 to 20 mg weekly. Careful monitoring of haematological and hepatic function is essential. The most likely side-effects are marrow depression and hepatic fibrosis. Marrow depression is rare at the usual doses, provided there are no adverse drug interactions, and liver damage is related to the cumulative total dose and to any past hepatic problems such as alcohol excess. Patients starting methotrexate should be counselled about avoiding or minimizing alcoholic intake while on methotrexate.

If long-term methotrexate use is envisaged, a pre-therapy liver biopsy should be considered as at present there are no non-invasive tests which give the equivalent information. This, however, has to be balanced against the fact that liver biopsy itself has a recognized morbidity and even mortality rate. Any patient who develops abnormal liver function tests while on methotrexate should have methotrexate discontinued, and the need for liver biopsy again be considered. Patients who are on long-term methotrexate should also be considered for liver biopsy when they reach a cumulative total dose of 1.5 g. Drug interactions are particularly important in patients on methotrexate. Non-steroidal anti-inflammatories, trimethoprim/sulphonamides, and systemic steroids are the main problems and concomitant therapy with these should be avoided in patients on methotrexate. Patients on methotrexate should carry a patient information sheet and drug interaction warning card.

Cyclosporin

Systemic cyclosporin is an effective method of controlling severe psoriasis. It is given orally at a dose of 2–4 mg/kg/day which can be reduced to a maintenance dose of 0.5–1 mg/kg/day as lesions clear. Initially, psoriatic plaques will clear rapidly, often within a week of starting treatment. However, psoriasis may return just as rapidly, when cyclosporin is withdrawn. This suggests that the mode of action, which is not yet understood, lies at a point close to expression of the psoriatic lesion. The assumption is that cyclosporin acts in psoriasis as an immunosuppressive agent, possibly by modifying T helper cell activity.

The main toxicity associated with cyclosporin is renal damage and full renal function studies should be carried out prior to commencing a patient on cyclosporin. Blood pressure, serum creatinine, and urea should be measured and two creatinine clearance tests should be carried out. While on cyclosporin, blood pressure serum creatinine and urea should be measured monthly, and creatinine clearance repeated 3–6 monthly. The dose of cyclosporin should be reduced or withdrawn if creatinine climbs more than 25 per cent above base line values and /or the diastolic blood pressure exceeds 95 mm Hg. Known drug interactions in the case of cyclosporin include aminoglycosides, trimethoprim, keto-conazole, phenytoin, rifampicin, isoniazid, and non-steroidal anti-inflammatories. Patients again should carry a patient information sheet and drug interaction warning.

Hydroxyurea

This drug is rarely used in the management of psoriasis, and would not normally be considered unless retinoids, cyclosporin, and methotrexate were inappropriate or treatment with these had failed. A 60 per cent improvement in 60 per cent of patients is reported. The dose is 1 g/day, and the main toxicities are bone marrow depression and teratogenicity. Patients on hydroxyurea, therefore, need regular haematological assessment and females must avoid pregnancy for 6 months after stopping the drug.

Systemic steroids

Very occasionally a short-term course of systemic steroids is the most appropriate treatment option in psoriasis. This could occur in otherwise uncontrollable erythroderma or extensive pustular psoriasis of the von Zumbush type.

Management of psoriasis of the nails and of psoriatic arthropathy

Severe nail involvement in psoriasis is difficult to treat, but nails may improve as cutaneous lesions are treated with for example PUVA. Psoriatic arthropathy may respond, at least in part, to systemic methotrexate or to cyclosporin, but patients with severe problems of both cutaneous and psoriatic arthropathy should be managed jointly by a dermatologist and rheumatologist. It is obviously very important to avoid severe drug interactions with systemic therapy used for cutaneous psoriasis, and non-steroidal anti-inflammatories prescribed for joint problems.

It can be seen that appropriate management of the patient with psoriasis requires careful initial consideration and constant reassessment to ensure that the treatment at that point in time is appropriate for the state of the patient's skin at that point.

The Psoriasis Association has branches in many countries and publishes useful literature for patients. Many psoriatics find membership of this Association of value.

Key Points

In lichen planus intensely itchy, flat-topped papules occur on the inner side of the wrists, lower legs, and mucous membranes.

Lichen planus

Definition

This is a purely cutaneous disorder with itchy, flat-topped papules most commonly seen on the inner surfaces of the wrists and the lower legs. The mucous membranes are usually affected. Spontaneous resolution usually takes place in a period of 3 months to 2 years.

Prevalence

This disease accounts for 0.2–0.8 per cent of dermatological outpatient consultations in Britain and North America.

Aetiology

The cause of lichen planus is unknown. A drug eruption virtually indistinguishable from so called idiopathic lichen planus can be precipitated by a wide variety of drugs, and the lesions of acute graft-versus-host disease are also very similar. This suggests that the problem has an underlying immunological basis. Lichen planus lesions can also be precipitated by trauma—the so called Koebner phenomenon.

Pathology

The pathology of lichen planus is that of the lichenoid tissue reaction, a pattern that is seen in a number of other conditions such as lichenoid drug eruptions. 'Liquefaction degeneration' or selective destruction of the basal layer of the epidermis gives the dermo–epidermal junction a ragged, 'saw-toothed' outline. A mixed cell infiltrate is seen in the papillary dermis. This infiltrate varies in density, but tends to be found in close contact with the overlying epidermis, and to contain some free melanin. Discrete round deposits of amorphous pink material may also be observed in the papillary dermis. These so-called 'colloid bodies' are thought to consist of disintegrating basal cells. There is a prominent, sometimes wedge-shaped, granular layer, and the epidermis is thinned in the atrophic and thickened in the hypertrophic form of the disease.

Immunofluorescence studies show large quantities of immunoglobulin on the colloid body surface. This is usually IgM and, although the resulting 'bunch of grapes' immunofluorescent pattern is striking, it is not diagnostic, as colloid bodies can be seen in a variety of states associated with basal cell degeneration.

Clinical features

Classically, the onset is acute with intensely itchy, red or violet, shiny, flat-topped papules. The flexor surfaces of wrists, the forearms and legs are the usual sites (Fig. 4.16). The oral mucous membrane is often affected at this time with white, spongy, slightly raised lesions, sometimes with a trabecular appearance, on the inner surfaces of the cheeks (Fig. 4.17). These lesions are commonly asymptomatic and unless specifically looked for, they may well be missed. They

Fig. 4.16 Lichen planus seen on the classic site of the inner wrist area. Note the bluish-red, flat-topped papule with an overlying white network. This pattern is referred to as Wickham's striae.

Fig. 4.17 Lichen planus of the oral mucous membranes. Note the white, web-line pattern on the inner surface of the cheek.

are, however, an important point in establishing the diagnosis. Similar lesions may be seen on the genitalia.

The cutaneous lesions may persist for many months, and characteristically develop a fine white network on their surface—a pattern called Wickham's striae. Pruritus generally tends to diminish in time. Rarer variants of lichen planus include:

- an annular or linear pattern
- atrophic
- ulcerative
- hypertrophic forms.

All of these tend to be more persistent and resistant to therapy than the classical type.

Involvement of the nails is seen in about 10 per cent of patients, usually those with the more chronic skin lesions. Fine ridging or grooving, severe dystrophy, and even complete destruction of the nail bed may occur.

Differential diagnosis

Lichen planus is normally fairly easily diagnosed on clinical grounds and histological confirmation is not always required. It is essential to take a good history to exclude the possibility of a lichenoid eruption due either to drugs (thiazides, antimalarials, and gold) or to external contact with photographic colour developers. Occasionally, when the clinical picture resembles psoriasis, biopsy will be required. Persistent ulcerative or hypertrophic lesions should also be biopsied to confirm the diagnosis.

Therapy

The most important aspect of treatment of lichen planus for the patient is control of itch. Moderately potent topical steroids are the most useful preparation and, for persistent itch, systemic sedating antihistamines may help. Stubborn lesions associated with severe and persistent itch may respond to intralesional steroid injections. Some dermatologists advocate a short course of systemic steroids for early severe cases, but the evidence that this is effective is lacking. There is no place for systemic steroid administration on a long-term basis or for chronic lesions.

Synthetic retinoids given systemically have been reported to be of benefit in some but not all studies of treatment of severe cutaneous or oral lichen planus and systemic cyclosporin A has also been reported of benefit in a few cases.

Pityriasis rosea

Definition

A self-limiting disorder characterized by the development of asymptomatic erythematous scaling macules on the trunk.

Key Points

Pityriasis rosea is self-limiting, usually affects the young, and causes asymptomatic, oval macules on the trunk, upper arms, and thighs.

Incidence and aetiology

Pityriasis rosea is most commonly seen in children and young adults. An increased incidence in spring and autumn, and outbreaks in institutions suggest that an infective agent, possibly viral, may be the aetiological agent.

Pathology

This is non-diagnostic and an accurate history and careful clinical examination are more reliable aids to diagnosis. If a biopsy is performed a moderately dense, mainly lymphocytic dermal infiltrate, papillary oedema, and a few extravasated red blood cells may be seen. Spongiosis may be seen in the epidermis at the edge of a developing lesion. This histological picture is very similar to that of secondary syphilis and, as the clinical picture may also be similar, the pathologist must be given an accurate clinical history or unfortunate confusion may arise. If there is any doubt, serology should be performed.

Clinical features

The first clinical lesion in pityriasis rosea is the herald patch, an isolated erythematous patch with a peripheral collarette of scale. This is usually seen on the trunk, up to a week before the main eruption appears and is followed by the development of oval macules, also with peripheral scaling, on the trunk, thighs, and upper arms. The trunk lesions tend to have their long axes parallel to the ribs, giving a so-called 'Christmas tree' distribution of the lesions (Fig. 4.18). Involvement of the hands, feet, or scalp is rare, and lesions are usually asymptomatic although there may be mild pruritus. Severe cases may have associated purpuric lesions.

Pityriasis rosea generally remits spontaneously in 4–8 weeks, but atypical or severe forms may be more persistent.

Fig. 4.18 Pityriasis rosea with typical involvement of the trunk. Secondary syphilis is an important differential diagnosis to consider.

Differential diagnosis

Secondary syphilis, drug eruptions, pityriasis versicolor, and occasionally guttate psoriasis must be considered. Serological studies will exclude syphilis and negative mycological examination will exclude pityriasis versicolor. A good history will eliminate a drug eruption and occasionally a biopsy may be required to rule out psoriasis.

Therapy

Once the diagnosis is established all that may be needed is reassurance of the benign and self-limiting nature of the disease. Troublesome itch can be relieved by a moderate potency topical steroid.

Pityriasis rubra pilaris

Definition

A rare erythematosquamous cutaneous eruption with characteristic follicular papules.

Incidence and aetiology

Pityriasis rubra pilaris (PRP) is uncommon. There are several clinical variants including a familial type with autosomal dominant inheritance. The cause is not yet known.

Pathology

There is hyperkeratosis, and parakeratosis around follicular openings, a mild inflammatory infiltrate in the papillary dermis, and apparent enlargement of the arrector pili muscles. This is a non-specific picture, and diagnosis should be based on clinical rather than on histological appearances.

Clinical features

In typical cases there is, on the trunk, a striking erythema in which occasional islands of normal skin can be seen. Follicular papules reminiscent of a nutmeg grater appear on the dorsa of the fingers, and a striking yellow-coloured hyper-keratosis develops on the palms and soles (Fig. 4.19). There are no symptoms and the patient is well. In general, spontaneous resolution occurs in 6 months to 2 years.

Differential diagnosis

Occasionally a biopsy will be needed to differentiate between PRP and either psoriasis or seborrhoeic dermatitis.

Therapy

This is difficult and unsatisfactory. A proportion of patients do well on acetretin (neotigason) 20–30 mg/day for 4 months or less if the condition resolves. Low doses of oral methotrexate 5–15 mg weekly may also be beneficial. Topical treatment with a keratolytic containing 2 per cent salicylic acid may be useful to help reduce hyperkeratosis of the palms and soles, and moderate potency topical steroid may reduce itch. PRP does not respond well to oral steroids.

Darier's disease

Definition

A genetically determined disease characterized by abnormal keratinization based mainly on the hair follicles and causing a greasy, reddish-brown papular eruption.

Aetiology

The gene for Darier's disease is situated on the long arm of chromosome 12, but the gene itself and its function have not yet been identified. The disease is transmitted by autosomal dominant inheritance, but as many patients have a negative family history, new mutations appear to be common.

Pathology

Abnormalities of keratinocytes are seen in the lower layers of the epidermis. Prematurely keratinized cells (corps ronds) and distorted keratinocyte nuclei ('grains') are seen causing parakeratosis.

Fig. 4.20 Darier's disease. The greasy papules on this young man's back appeared for the first time as a severe episode of sunburn was fading from the mid-zone of his trunk.

Fig. 4.21 Nails and Darier's disease showing striking nicking at the free margin.

Clinical features

Darier's disease is usually first seen in young adults as greasy brown papules on the chest and scapular area. It may be aggravated by sunlight and may have an acute onset after sunburn (Fig. 4.20). Small pits on the skin of the palm of the hand and irregular nicks at the distal end of the nails are also present (Fig. 4.21). Cutaneous infections with herpes simplex may give rise to very severe widespread infection—so-called Kaposi's varicelliform eruption in patients with Darier's disease, suggesting that they have a localized immune defect.

Treatment

Some patients with very mild Darier's disease may require no specific treatment. For others with the more severe forms of the disease acetretin (Neotigason) 20 mg/day is very effective. As with the treatment of severe psoriasis with retinoids, caution must be taken to ensure that the drug is not given to pregnant women, and that contraception is maintained for a minimum of two years after stopping the drug because of teratogenicity and a long half-life of acetretin. Cheilitis is a common minor side-effect and temporary elevation of triglycerides may occur, particularly if the patient is obese.

Moderate potency topical steroids for itch, and salicylic acid preparations to reduce scaling have largely been superseded by the retinoids.

The Ichthyoses

Definition

Disorders of keratinization, usually genetically determined, characterized by excessively dry and visibly scaly skin:

- autosomal dominant ichthyosis vulgaris
- X-linked recessive ichthyosis
- bullous ichthyosiform erythroderma (epidermolytic hyperkeratosis).

The majority of patients with ichthyosis present in infancy and childhood. The remainder acquire the condition in adolescence or adult life. It has been reported in some series that a proportion of patients with adult-onset ichthyosis may have an underlying neoplasm, usually of haematological origin.

Autosomal dominant ichthyosis vulgaris

In the UK, autosomal dominant ichthyosis is common, having a prevalence of 1 in 250 to 1 in 300. There is an underlying disorder of keratinization seen on light microscopy as an absent epidermal granular layer.

Clinical features

Affected children present in early childhood with a rough, dry skin, most marked on the extensor surfaces of the arms and worst in winter. The scales are fine and white. Many children have rough, horny papules, seen best on the extensor surfaces of the upper arms, thought to be due to faulty keratinization around hair follicle openings (Fig. 4.22). The skin of patients with atopic dermatitis is dry, but the relationship of this xerosis (dry skin) to true ichthyosis is uncertain. Dominant ichthyosis vulgaris tends to improve slowly during childhood and puberty, but may also persist into adult life.

Treatment

This depends on the use of lubricants and emulsifying preparations. Excessive use of soap should be discouraged, and emulsifying ointment BP substituted. Water-soluble oils should be added to bath-water or used after bathing. Preparations containing urea in a water-miscible base may help to maintain adequate hydration of the stratum corneum, (for example Calmurid) but some patients complain of intense stinging for a few minutes after their application. Topical steroids should not be used routinely to lubricate dry skin.

Sex-linked recessive ichthyosis (ichthyosis nigricans)

Prevalence and aetiology

This is very much rarer than the autosomal dominant variety and, although the fully developed disease is seen in males only, female heterozygotes may have mild degrees of the condition, mainly on the lower legs. An associated abnormality is a deficiency of the enzyme steroid sulphatase seen in both affected children and carrier mothers. This enzyme deficiency can be detected in the placenta but does not appear to be associated with any increased incidence of perinatal problems although affected mothers may give a history of excessively long labours.

Fig. 4.22 Autosomal dominant ichthyosis. Fine, white scales are most profuse on the upper arms.

Pathology

There is a striking increase in the granular layer with a thickened overlying stratum corneum.

Clinical features

There are large, greasy, polygonal, yellow or brown scales mainly on the trunk (Fig. 4.23). There is little tendency for the condition to improve with time. Removing the scales with abrasion and copious emollients are the usual methods of controlling the disease. Use of systemic retinoids has produced conflicting reports, but gene transfer is a possible future approach.

Bullous ichthyosiform erythroderma

A rare disorder in which patients have both erythrodermatous skin and blisters in varying combinations. This condition is inherited by autosomal dominant transmission, and is caused by mutations in the genes for keratins 1 and 10.

Biopsy of affected skin shows very characteristic blister formation within the epidermis, even if the area chosen for biopsy is not clinically bullous. Affected babies usually have extensive blistering and desquamation at birth, sometimes giving rise to fluid balance problems. In later life scaling on an erythematous base predominates.

Treatment

Liberal use of emollients is the best approach. Oral retinoids have again not been uniformly successful.

Other very rare ichthyotic conditions include those with systemic associations such as Refsum's syndrome, due to a specific defect in phytanic acid metabolism and characterized by ichthyosis, retinitis pigmentosa, and neurological defects.

Fig. 4.23 Ichthyosis nigricans (sex-linked ichthyosis vulgaris). The scales are large, greasy and yellowish in colour.

Discussion of problem cases (see pp. 43–4)

Case 4.1

The important points in this woman's history are, firstly, that she wishes a cosmetically acceptable method of controlling her psoriasis, and, secondly, that this remedy must not be teratogenic in view of her wish to conceive. At her age, time is not on her side.

In general, in younger adults, it is preferable to try to control psoriasis with topical treatment as all systemic approaches to psoriasis management have some toxicity. PUVA can give rise to cutaneous malignancies, methotrexate is toxic to the liver, and cyclosporin can cause renal toxicity. All of these complications are related to the cumulative total dose, so starting systemic treatment of any type as late in life as possible makes sense in the case of a chronic relapsing and remitting disease. None of the above systemic agents are safe for use in young women of child bearing potential who are not taking full contraceptive precautions, usually the oral contraceptive.

Oral retinoids are less toxic to the patient him or herself long term, but are absolutely ruled out in this woman's case as they are potent teratogens. In addition, they are stored in the body fat for as long as 2 years after discontinuation of oral administration, so if a 36 year old were given a retinoid she could not even attempt to conceive until she was 38 whether or not this successfully cleared her psoriasis.

We, therefore, come to the choices of topical therapy in various combinations with or without added UVB therapy. Topical tar is effective, but messy to apply, and the cleaner proprietary tars tend to be less effective. Topical dithranol is effective, but may irritate surrounding normal skin and must therefore be used with care. Calcipotriol or calcipotriene is moderately effective but rarely removes all traces of psoriasis.

Any of these 3 preparations can also be used in association with UVB radiation therapy. Current evidence suggests that the use of narrow band UVB therapy in the 310 to 312 nanometre (nm) range is more effective than broader band UV and has less risk of long-term side effects, particularly carcinogenesis, as lower cumulative total doses are needed.

Our patient wants a full discussion of the possible treatment options including a full explanation as to why none of the 'psoriasis pills' are appropriate for her. She opted for a weak concentration of proprietary dithranol (0.25 per cent with gradually increasing concentrations to 1.0 per cent dithocream). This was applied as short-contact dithranol with the patient using it for 20 to 30 minutes each morning before showering and dressing for work. In addition, she had a 6 week course of narrow band UVB therapy, attending 3 times a week after work at the local outpatient treatment centre. On this regime her psoriasis cleared well and remained clear for the next 4 months during which she had a 2 week Mediterranean holiday which was almost certainly of additional value in maintaining her clearance.

Six months later she returned with mild psoriasis and 8 weeks pregnant. Her psoriasis remained virtually clear throughout pregnancy, quite a common observation, but flared again 6 weeks after delivery. A further course of UVB at the local out-patient treatment centre cleared the lesions and did not interfere with breast feeding.

She asks you about the chances that her son will develop psoriasis. How will you reply?

Case 4.2

This elderly gentleman lives alone and the nearest dermatology out-patient treatment centre is 20 miles away. His psoriasis is seriously affecting his ability to continue to live independently and his arthritis makes it very difficult for him to use topical treatments. Possible approaches here would include:

1. Regular (daily or 3 to 4 times a week) topical applications with help from the local district nurse or practice nurse.

2. Systemic treatment with retinoids, methotrexate, or cyclosporin A.

Initially, a trial of district nurse management was conducted. She came in 3 times a week to help in applying first weak tar and then calcipotriol. However, on both of these routines, his psoriasis flared and became irritable. Topical, moderate potency steroids were also tried but also with little benefit. After some discussion, the patient was then given a 6 week trial of oral methotrexate, 10 mg weekly, once it had been established that his liver function was normal and his creatinine clearance adequate for his age. He was counselled to avoid all alcohol while he was taking methotrexate. His psoriasis cleared within 3 weeks on this regime with no elevation of liver function tests, or serum creatinine, or fall in white cell count. His arthropathy also improved to the extent that he planned his first holiday in 6 years. He continues to take his oral methotrexate 10 mg orally weekly under district nurse supervision, attends the general practitioner monthly for liver function tests and white cell counts, and sees his local consultant dermatologist quarterly.

1. What advice **must** this patient be given about drug interactions and methotrexate?

2. What specific investigation should be considered as a base line in patients in whom you are contemplating methotrexate therapy long term?

3. What are the risks and benefits of carrying out this particular investigation?

Case 4.3

While the description of the lesions might suggest insect bites, they do not usually last as long as 6 weeks. Again, the timing and duration of therapy do not suggest that a drug eruption is a likely diagnosis. The site of the lesions and the itch both suggest lichen planus as a possible diagnosis. On examination, the patient had white patches in her mouth. A small punch biopsy was taken from the wrist and showed a lichenoid tissue reaction, compatible with a diagnosis of lichen planus. The lesions cleared slowly over the next 5 months during which moderate potency topical steroids were prescribed.

Case 4.4

The history here suggests the possibility of impetigo complicating severe sunburn, or possibly secondary viral infection on pre-existing eczema. However, there is no past personal or family history of eczema.

Swabs were taken for bacteriological and viral culture, and the young man started on topical and systemic antistaphylococcal antibiotics. Two days later the virologists reported a heavy growth of herpes simplex type 1, and he was started on full doses of systemic acyclovir. The infection cleared rapidly, leaving raised papules on his back. A biopsy of one of these showed disruption of the epidermis with grains and corps ronds. This pattern is diagnostic of Darier's disease. Darier's disease appears frequently for the first time after sun damage, and is a condition associated with severe secondary h. simplex infection or Kaposi's varicelliform eruption. What other signs might this young man have?

Case 4.5

Review this history carefully. It does not suggest psoriasis. Psoriasis can begin in infancy but this is unusual without a positive family history, and with no response to normally effective antipsoriatic therapy. A biopsy should be carried out.

The biopsy showed none of the features of psoriasis, but the presence in the mid epidermis of swollen keratinocytes, a characteristic pathological feature of bullous ichthyosiform erythroderma. Clinically, bullae are often only seen in infancy, and in older children and adults extensive erythroderma with fine white scales is more common. The patient was treated with copious emollients with moderate benefit.

Always carefully review a long-standing diagnosis if there is a poor response to seemingly appropriate treatment.

Projects

1. Ask the next six people with psoriasis who you see in general practice, in the outpatient department treatment centre, or in the dermatology ward for 5 minutes of their time. Prepare a brief 2 page questionnaire asking how **they** feel about their psoriasis, and how this has affected their lives. Include questions on family problems, difficult situations at work, on holidays, on relationships with the opposite sex and possible problems relating to the hairdresser and buying clothes. Ask them if there was a complete cure for psoriasis how much they would be willing to pay for this. Relate the sum they quote to their life-style and apparent income.

   What are the common features amongst the six people, and what has this study told you about psoriasis and disability?

   Could any of the points brought up by the six patients you have spoken to be relevant to any other dermatological conditions?

2. Make a list of the systemic drugs used in the management of patients with psoriasis. Draw up an appropriate information and drug interaction warning card for patients who are on each of these systemic therapies to carry. Think carefully about any necessary regular

investigations and how often these should be done. If you were the general practitioner of patients on these drugs what specific points would you look for in the letter from the local dermatologist.

Further reading

Camisa, C. (1994). *Psoriasis.* Blackwell Scientific Oxford.

An excellent source of information on both clinical and basic scientific aspects of psoriasis.

Roenigk, H.H. and Maibach, H.I. (ed.) (1990). *Psoriasis* (2nd edn). Marcel Dekker, New York.

Another excellent source of detailed information.

British Association of Dermatologists (1995). *Guidelines for the management of patients with psoriasis.*

Dermatitis and eczema

- The terms dermatitis and eczema

- Mechanisms of cutaneous inflammation

- Acute, subacute, and chronic dermatitis

- Atopic dermatitis

- Nummular or discoid dermatitis

- Asteatoric eczema (eczema craquelé)

- Seborrhoeic dermatitis

- Contact dermatitis

- Patient association

The varieties of eczema and dermatitis which will be discussed in this chapter are:

- atopic dermatitis
- nummular dermatitis (discoid dermatitis)
- asteatotic eczema (eczema craquelé)
- seborrhoeic dermatitis
- contact dermatitis: direct irritant—including napkin dermatitis: allergic contact dermatitis
- dishydrotic eczema (pompholyx)
- neurodermatitis (circumscribed lichen simplex)
- prurigo nodularis
- stasis dematitis

Problem cases

Case 5.1

A young couple come to see you together to ask for your help in treating their first child, a boy now aged 9 months, who has had red apparently itchy skin since the age of three months. He was exclusively breast fed until the age of 4 months but is now on mixed feeding including cows milk. He is very irritable, sleeps badly, and scratches continually. His parents say they are desperate. What is the likely diagnosis, are any investigations required, and how would you manage the child?

Case 5.2

A 28-year-old postdoctoral scientist in your local University consults you about persistent dandruff, sticky eyes, a rash in the nasolabial fold, and a vague generalized itch. He is very concerned about scabies. What diagnosis does this presentation suggest and what is your management plan?

Case 5.3

An 18-year-old hairdresser consults you about dry, scaly patches on the dorsum of her hands which have developed over the past year. She started hairdressing 2 years ago, and has a past history of asthma as a child. She herself blames the perm lotion which comes into contact with her skin although she wears rubber gloves most of the time. What is the likely diagnosis and what investigations and treatment are indicated?

Case 5.4

A 69-year-old, obese, retired teacher consults you about dermatitis around her right ankle with obvious underlying varicose veins. The skin is red, irritable, and inflamed. She has been applying a cream to it given to her by her sister, but thinks that this may have made the problem worse. What investigations and treatment might be appropriate here?

Suggested diagnoses and treatment plans will be found on p. 104.

The terms dermatitis and eczema

The term dermatitis simply means inflammation of the skin and can be qualified according to the likely cause, while the term eczema has no clear universally agreed definition. In the past, there has been a suggestion that one could think of this group of disorders as either exogenous—due to an obvious external cause, or endogenous—no obvious external cause and assumed to be due to genetic susceptibility. This led to the idea that the term eczema should be used to describe endogenous problems, and dermatitis for exogenous problems. Nowadays, however, this distinction has become blurred as we understand better, for example, the interaction between exogenous and endogenous factors in atopy. For these reasons most dermatologists prefer the term dermatitis rather than eczema to describe this group of disorders, qualified by the type of dermatitis, as it is simply and clearly defined as inflammation of the skin, and the pathological appearance is also well established.

Mechanisms of cutaneous inflammation

Cell marker studies have established that the T lymphocyte is preferentially recruited into the dermis and epidermis in the great majority of cutaneous inflammatory processes, and in most situations the CD4$^+$ helper T lymphocyte is found in much larger numbers than the CD8$^+$ T cytotoxic or suppressor subset. In patients with atopic dermatitis the majority of these T helper lymphocytes are of the TH2 subset, (see p. 80).

If timed sequential biopsies are carried out of skin on which inflammation has been deliberately induced, polymorphonuclear leukocytes will be found about 4–6 hours after applying the inflammatory stimulus. By 24 hours, virtually all the cells present are lymphocytes. Both lymphocyte function associated antigen (LFA) and gamma interferon are also expressed in the epidermis and on cells in the papillary dermis early in the dermatitis reaction. The role of tumour necrosis factor alpha in these interactions is also currently under investigation.

The role of the Langerhans cell in the inflammatory reaction in the skin, and particularly in the induction of allergic contact dermatitis, is now partly understood. Langerhans cells can function as antigen-presenting cells, although they are not as efficient as macrophages. Potentially antigenic materials absorbed through the skin become bound to the surface of Langerhans cells which can then traffic in the lymphatic system to the local draining lymph nodes where the development of a specifically sensitized clone of lymphocytes takes place. What is not understood is the reason why any one contact with, for example, nickel results in sensitization and subsequent contact dermatitis, while many other apparently identical events, both in other individuals and in the patient himself prior to his developing dermatitis, do not.

Acute, subacute, and chronic dermatitis

Dermatitis of any of the clinical varieties discussed below may be acute, subacute, or chronic. Each of these three stages has distinct clinical and pathological appearances. It is necessary to be able to identify these three phases or stages in the dermatitis reaction as they all require different approaches to treatment. At any time, one lesion on a patient may be acute, while a second lesion on another part of the body may be subacute or even chronic. This is particularly true of atopic dermatitis.

Acute dermatitis is inflamed oedematous oozing epidermis, which is seen on biopsy as an area of gross oedema within the epidermis, pushing individual keratinocytes apart, and thus causing the development of vesicles or small blisters.

Subacute dermatitis is the presence of visible scale and crust associated with inflamed skin, and here on biopsy one sees the scaling and crusting and also the epidermal disruption with a lymphocytic infiltrate among these keratinocytes.

Chronic dermatitis is seen as a thickened, often purple or violaceous, elevated plaque, and this on biopsy is seen as epidermal acanthosis or thickening with a lymphocytic infiltrate in the papillary dermis.

Table 5.1 outlines the features of acute, subacute, and chronic dermatitis.

Atopic dermatitis

Definition

A chronic extremely itchy form of dermatitis with a strong genetic aetiological component, often beginning in infancy and frequently associated with asthma and rhinitis.

Prevalence and aetiology

Atopic dermatitis currently affects 1–3 per cent of all infants in the UK. In later childhood and in adults the incidence is lower. Children with atopic dermatitis form a high proportion of those attending paediatric dermatology clinics. In certain ethnic groups, such as the Chinese, it seems to be rarer, but more severe and persistent than in Caucasians. Cohort studies of children born in the UK

Key Points

Atopic patients are prone to severe herpes simplex type 1 infection.

Table 5.1.

Clinical and pathological features of the acute, subacute, and chronic phases of the dermatitis reaction

	Acute	Subacute	Chronic
Clinical	Redness, swelling, oozing	Redness, swelling, crusting	Scaling. Thickening of the skin
	Formation of small blisters	Scaling, secondary infection	and increase in skin
	Pain, heat, tenderness	Itch—may be severe	markings—lichenification. Itch
Pathological	Dermal and epidermal oedema (spongiosis)	Crusting and parakeratosis	Scaling, parakeratosis
	Dilated and congested dermal capillaries	Early acanthosis	Marked acanthosis (epidermal thickening)
	Dermal infiltrate very early	Oedema	Coarsening of papillary dermal
	leucocytes, later lymphocytes	Perivascular lymphocytic dermal infiltrate	collagen
		Few lymphocytes also in dermis	

over the last 20 years show that the incidence and prevalence of all types of atopic disease are rising. The reason for this increase is not yet known.

Most patients with atopic dermatitis have a positive family history of the atopic triad—dermatitis, asthma, and allergic rhinitis. Although the exact mode of inheritance is obscure, autosomal dominance with variable penetration is postulated. One large study has associated the area around chromosome 11q13 with respiratory atopy but this has not yet been confirmed for cutaneous atopy.

Serum levels of immunoglobulin E are elevated in 80 per cent, but within the normal range in the remaining 20 per cent of patients with atopic dermatitis. Conversely about 5 per cent of the normal population have elevated IgE levels but are clinically normal. Thus, an elevated IgE level is neither necessary nor sufficient for a diagnosis of atopic dermatitis.

The results of *radioallergosorbent* testing (RAST) to determine the specific antigens against which IgE is synthesized differ in infants and older children. In infants, high RAST levels will be found against foods—usually eggs, dairy products, and fish. At around one year of age the pattern changes, and the bulk of the elevated IgE is directed against inhaled allergens such as the house dust mite (*D. pteronissinus*), animal hair, and pollens.

Our current understanding of the complex immunological abnormalities observed in patients with atopic dermatitis suggests the there is a disorder of immune regulation involving an imbalance in number and function of T cell subsets. T helper lymphocytes can be divided into TH1 and TH2 subsets, and in atopic dermatitis there is over activity of the TH2 subset. These lymphocytes produce interleukin 4 and interleukin 5, which in turn stimulate IgE production by B lymphocytes. In contrast, the numbers and activity of TH1 lymphocytes is low. TH1 lymphocytes stimulate production of gamma interferon and the fact that the cord blood levels of gamma interferon are low in babies born to atopic mothers, and who subsequently develop atopic dermatitis themselves, suggests that this could be a primary rather than a secondary immunological event in the development of atopic dermatitis. These low levels of gamma interferon may be due to increased activity of cyclic AMP phosphodiesterase which cause increased synthesis of prostaglandin E2 which in turn inhibits gamma interferon production, thus perpetuating a cycle of over-activity. These observations have stimulated the experimental use of gamma interferon in atopic dermatitis therapy (see p. 87).

In atopic dermatitis there are also vascular abnormalities as the cutaneous vasculature responds abnormally to stimulation. Instead of a normal 'weal and flare' response, firm rubbing of the skin elicits **white dermographism** as a simple white linear streak along the site of pressure with no erythema.

Clinical features

Sixty percent of those who have atopic dermatitis first develop it in infancy. It may appear as early as 6 weeks, with apparently itchy scaly lesions on the scalp, face, and trunk. The infant will be irritable, restless, and wakeful and tries to rub the affected areas. In babies the cheeks, wrists, and hands are usually red, scaling, and scratched, but even in severe disease there may be sparing of the central panel of the face (Fig. 5.1).

In toddlers and older children, the common sites of involvement are the elbow, knee, and buttock flexures, the ankles, the dorsa of the feet under straps of shoes, the retroauricular fold, and the antecubital fossae (Fig. 5.2). In severe cases there may be extensive involvement of all four limbs with gross excoriation and secondary infection.

In about 80 per cent of affected children atopic dermatitis clears spontaneously between the ages of 2 and 5 years, but if it continues into adoles-

Fig. 5.1 Atopic dermatitis in infancy. The face and scalp are often affected in young children, and relative sparing of the perioral and nasal region is common as seen here.

Fig. 5.2 Atopic dermatitis involving the knee flexures lichenification and recent excoriations.

Fig. 5.3 Severe atopic dermatitis in an adult. Note gross lichenification and superimposed excoriations.

cence and adult life it enters the chronic phase with striking lichenification in the popliteal and antecubital fossae and on the nape of the neck (Fig. 5.3). Prominent infraorbital creases are also seen, giving a weary and prematurely aged expression. Thinning of the lateral half of the eyebrows (Hertoghe's sign) is frequently present, due to continual rubbing. Shiny fingernails result from buffing rather than scratching the lesions.

Adults with atopic dermatitis tend to have a generalized dry skin associated with diffuse, itchy plaques involving large areas of the trunk and face.

A mild degree of ichthyosis and 'keratosis pilaris' may also be present. This consists of horny papules of the orifices of the hair follicles, and is most easily seen and felt on the outer surface of the upper arm.

Asthma may coexist and may either be very active at the same time as the skin, or flare independently.

Atopic dermatitis and contact dermatitis

Large studies suggest that patients with atopic dermatitis have a lower incidence of allergic contact dermatitis, but are more susceptible than non-atopics to irritant contact dermatitis. It is most important, therefore, to offer atopic adolescents guidance about careers and to indicate those occupations which are inadvisable. Many atopic girls are interested in a nursing career because of their knowledge of hospital life, but this should not be encouraged as continual exposure to soap and water causes exacerbation of hand lesions. Many student nurse training programmes will not take individuals with a past history of atopic dermatitis for this reason.

Investigations

No specific investigations are usually required to confirm the diagnosis in patients with atopic dermatitis and the diagnosis should be made on clinical grounds. As stated above, not all patients with atopic dermatitis have a raised

IgE so a normal level will not exclude the diagnosis. Blood should not be taken routinely from infants with suspected atopic dermatitis as IgE levels are usually within the normal range until after 6 months, even if the infant has severe dermatitis.

Prick tests to a wide range of allergens can be carried out on older children and adults but they tend to confirm what is already known on history, and again are not recommended as a therapeutically useful routine investigation. They can be very distressing to young children.

Bacteriological swabs taken from affected areas of skin will usually show a heavy growth of *Staphylococcus aureus*, but again this is non-specific, and it may be difficult to decide if this is simple secondary bacterial colonization, which will clear with routine treatment, or if specific antistaphylococcal therapy is needed.

A test which may be of therapeutic relevance in patients with vesicles and suspected atopic dermatitis or with an unexplained exacerbation of pre-existing atopic dermatitis is to swab the skin for herpes simplex virus. Atopic patients are prone to severe herpes simplex type 1 infections (see below), and this requires antiviral therapy.

Complications and associations (Table 5.2)

The most important complication of atopic dermatitis is the development of eczema herpeticum or Kaposi's varicelliform eruption after exposure to herpes simplex type 1 virus. This is seen as the presence of small blisters in areas of dermatitis and general malaise with fever. This can cause severe systemic upset which prior to the availability of acyclovir could be fatal. It is, therefore, very

Table 5.2.
Problems associated with atopic dermatitis

Dermatological

Severe infection with herpes simplex type 1—eczema herpeticum

Increased colonization of the epidermis by *Staphylococcus aureus*

Dry skin—either xerosis of atopy, or autosomal dominant ichthyosis

Dry and prominent hair follicles, particularly on upper arms—keratosis pilaris

Juvenile plantar dermatosis; shiny, tender soles of feet with tendency to fissure formation

In female adults, nipple dermatitis

Increased incidence of persistent and stubborn warts and *Molluscum contagiosum*

Ocular

Cataract and keratoconus

Gastrointestinal

Food intolerance and food allergy

Fig. 5.4 Patient with atopic dermatitis and Kaposi's varicelliform eruption. Note striking eruption on forehead.

Fig. 5.5 Kaposi's varicelliform eruption in a 3-year-old child with mild atopic dermatitis. Herpes simplex virus was isolated from the lesions.

important that parents of children with atopic dermatitis know that their child should not come into contact with individuals who have simple cold sores, as atopic children are at risk of a much more extensive and serious herpes simplex infection (Figs 5.4, 5.5, and 5.6).

Diet and atopic dermatitis

The relationship between food allergy or intolerance and atopic dermatitis is controversial. In a small proportion of patients certain specific foods, most commonly dairy products and eggs, appear to cause an exacerbation of the disease. This is usually seen in children, and there is little evidence that food allergies cause or exacerbate atopic dermatitis in the majority of older children and adults.

Treatment

The start of management of the atopic patient or the parent of an atopic child is to explain the nature of the disease, and that control rather than cure is the aim. It is reasonable, however, to be optimistic concerning spontaneous regression, particularly in the case of young children.

The manner in which treatment prescribed are used is extremely important in atopic eczema, and if at all possible patients should have a demonstration of how to apply their topical application and how to use bandages from a trained dermatological nurse. This can be done in an out-patient centre, health centre, or, best of all, in the patients own home.

The following treatments are useful for patients with mild and moderate dermatitis:

- emollients
- topical steroids
- sedating antihistamines
- antibiotics
- wet wrap dressings
- ichthyol impregnated bandages
- ultraviolet light (UVB)
- environmental change

For more severe cases the following treatments may be required:

- evening primrose oil—Efamol
- photochemotherapy (PUVA)
- cyclosporin
- Azathioprine
- experimental therapy—gamma interferon and thymic extracts
- alternative medicine approaches—Chinese herbs and hypnotherapy
- Acyclovir for superimposed herpes simplex infections

Emollients

Most patients with atopic dermatitis have a dry skin and appropriate use of emollients can greatly reduce discomfort and itch. They can also reduce the quantity and potency of topical steroids needed. Preparations such as emulsifying ointment BP, or 50 per cent liquid paraffin in white soft paraffin should be used in place of soap to prevent further drying. Emollients can be prescribed for use both in and after the bath or shower. A wide range is available, and it is useful to initially prescribe small quantities of several preparations with different textures so that the patient can find what suits him best. Bath additives include Hydromol, Emulsiderm, and Oilatum; after bath preparations include Ung Merck and aqueous cream BP. It is wise to try to use emollients which are lanolin, preservative, and fragrance free to avoid the risk of sensitization. The addition of urea to emollients in preparations such as aquadrate and calmurid may increase their efficacy, but some children and adults find they cause quite severe stinging.

Topical steroids

Weak and moderately potent topical steroids are of great value in the regular management of atopic dermatitis. It is, however, important not to prescribe them for long periods of time without regular clinical review to see if the steroid potency can be reduced. Patients should be taught that while red skin needs some topical steroid, dry skin needs only an emollient. Care should be taken not to use steroids more potent than 1 per cent hydrocortisone on the face for longer than 1–2 weeks without review, as it is usually the thin skin of the face that is first to show the atrophy and telangiectasia associated with topical steroid overuse. It is also important to avoid over prescription of topical steroids in children to avoid both topical and systemic side-effects which can occur as a result of absorption of topical steroids through inflamed skin.

Fig. 5.6 Same child in Fig. 5.3, 3 months later. Note complete healing and absence of scarring.

Antibiotics

The combination of a topical steroid and antistaphylococcal antibiotic is often useful as staphylococcal infection can aggravate atopic dermatitis, and treating the staphylococcal colonization is frequently associated with clinical improvement. The antibiotic can be used either as a topical steroid antibiotic combination (for example fucidin hydrocortisone) or a single topical agent for example mupirocin, or given orally as a 5 day course of flucloxacillin or other appropriate antibiotic based on bacteriological sensitivity. There is currently some concern about the emergence of methicillin resistant staphylococci so, as with topical steroids, patients should be reviewed regularly, and a course of antibiotics should not continue indefinitely.

Antihistamines

Sedating antihistamines will help control the itch of atopic dermatitis and prevent night time scratching, but the more modern non-sedating antihistamines are of less benefit. Promethazine and trimeprazine are both useful and should be used alternately as patients tend to become used to one preparation after 3–4 weeks.

Wet wraps

This term describes the use of a damp stockinet suit held in place by a dry suit with either a weak antiseptic, such as Burrows solution (aluminium acetate), or a diluted topical steroid in contact with the skin. This is easiest to use at night and the beneficial effect is probably a combination of good hydration, the therapeutic affect of the chosen application, and the fact that two layers of stockinet make scratching very difficult. The technique is mainly used for short periods of time for small children and infants, and care must be taken to avoid hypothermia.

Occlusive bandaging

The use of ichthyol impregnated bandages (ichthopaste) over a topical steroid is also useful in preventing scratching and keeping the steroid in contact with the skin for the maximum amount of time. They can be left in place for 48 hours or longer. This technique is particularly useful for stubborn lesions on the limbs.

Ultraviolet B irradiation

Many patients with atopic dermatitis find that their skin improves greatly in sunny weather, and the majority also benefit from a 6 week course of UVB given three times weekly. Current work suggests that narrow band UVB using light in the 310–312 nm range is extremely effective.

Environmental change

It is sensible to try to reduce allergen exposure as far as is compatible with leading a fairly normal life. The house dust mite collects in carpets curtains and bedding, so a wooden floor, blinds in place of curtains and a non-permeable cover for the mattress and quilt may all help as will keeping the environment at a relatively low level of temperature and humidity. Hair bearing pets should be discouraged, and clothing should be of cotton rather than wool, which can be very irritant.

The management of severe atopic dermatitis

Treatments suggested below should only be considered when the more established methods suggested above have failed. Remember that although atopic dermatitis is distressing, it is benign. Many of the treatments discussed below have potentially serious side-effects and should not be used without thoughtfully balancing the risk/ benefit ratio, particularly in young children.

Gamolenic acid (Epogam)

There are conflicting opinions on the value of epogam or evening primrose oil in atopic dermatitis. To date, no specific abnormality of fatty acid metabolism requiring correction has been identified in atopic dermatitis patients, but a small proportion do appear to benefit. If patients wish a trial of epogam therapy, it is important to give an adequate dose of 12 capsules a day (480 mg) for an adult and 8 (320 mg) for a child. If there is no benefit after 6–8 weeks treatment the epogam should be withdrawn.

Dietary restriction

Many parents and some patients have the impression that their atopic dermatitis is exacerbated or caused by certain foods. These are usually dairy products, eggs, fish, and nuts. Dietary exclusion is rarely effective in atopic dermatitis, but if the patient is enthusiastic and able to cooperate, a time limited trial of elimination of certain foods is worth considering. The assistance of a qualified dietician is essential, particularly in the case of children, to ensure that the remaining diet is adequate, particularly in calcium intake. The best trial of dietary treatment is total compliance and rigorous exclusion of specific foods in rotation for 4–6 weeks. The diet should be stopped if there is no benefit.

Photochemotherapy—PUVA

Patients with severe atopic dermatitis may benefit from a 4–6 weeks course of PUVA treatment to clear recalcitrant atopic dermatitis. However, it is very important to keep a careful note of the cumulative total dose of UVA as there is now clear evidence that PUVA does increase the risk of non-melanoma skin cancer, and that this risk is related to the total dose of UVA. Maintenance PUVA should not be used to control atopic dermatitis for this reason.

Cyclosporin

The immunosuppressive drug cyclosporin (Neoral or Sandimmun) is extremely effective in controlling severe atopic dermatitis. However, high doses usually in the 2–5 mg/kg/day range are needed, and these may cause renal toxicity. If a patient has atopic dermatitis of a severity requiring consideration for cyclosporin treatment, two creatinine clearance studies should be carried out, and blood pressure, serum urea, and creatinine monitored regularly while on treatment. A 6–8 week course of treatment which can be repeated is recommended. Elevation of creatinine levels 25 per cent or more above baseline levels should be an indication for withdrawal of cyclosporin. Low dose maintenance treatment has been suggested, but results are not always satisfactory.

Azathioprine

The cytotoxic drug azathioprine or imuran will also control atopic dermatitis. Doses of 50–100 mg/day are usually effective, but patients must be monitored carefully for marrow depression and hepatic damage.

Experimental therapy—Gamma interferon and thymic extracts

As already discussed, patients with atopic dermatitis have an imbalance of T cell function and poor production of gamma interferon. One double blind controlled trial of gamma interferon 50 μg/m^2 injections daily for 12 weeks showed benefit. Despite the theory of TH1/TH2 imbalance, treatment with gamma interferon has not to date been associated with a fall in elevated IgE.

Thymopentin, an active extract of thymic hormone, has also been given by injection with some benefit, on the basis that the immunological abnormality underlying atopic dermatitis is a delayed maturation of the immune system.

Alternative or complementary medicine—Chinese herbal therapy and hypnotherapy

A randomized double blind study has shown benefit in patients with diffuse widespread atopic dermatitis when given a decoction of a particular blend of chinese herbs. The active ingredients have not been identified, but a corticosteroid effect has been excluded. Patients who wish to use chinese herbs should have liver function checked regularly as hepatotoxocity has been reported. A modified extract of chinese herbs, Zemaphyte, is currently available in the UK on a named patient basis, but there are as yet few reports of its efficacy.

Management of eczema herpeticum

Always consider the diagnosis of eczema herpeticum in any atopic dermatitis patient who develops vesicles, or who shows rapid deterioration, particularly if there is systemic upset. Swabs and blister fluid should be taken for virus identification and the patient should be commenced on systemic acyclovir without waiting for laboratory results. If the patient is febrile, acyclovir should be given intravenously for the first 28–72 hours at a dose of 5 mg/kg/day for adults. Topical steroids should not be applied to the infected skin.

Conclusion

This long list of possible approaches to atopic dermatitis control clearly indicates that at present there is no reliable, proven, effective, and safe method of permanently suppressing symptoms. Fortunately, in the great majority of patients, the condition is self limiting and clears spontaneously by the age of 5 years. For older patients the prognosis must be more guarded.

Nummular or discoid dermatitis

Definition

A chronic, recurrent pattern of dermatitis with discrete coin-shaped lesions tending to involve the limbs.

Incidence and aetiology

This variety of dermatitis usually affects adults, many of whom will have a past history of atopic dermatitis. The aetiology is unknown and, although secondary infection is common, a primary infective cause has not been proven.

Clinical features

The lesions are circular, ranging from 4 to 10 cm or more in diameter and are often distributed symmetrically on the legs (Fig. 5.7). They are usually subacute with erythema, mild oedema, and, in some cases, vesiculation. The surface may be moist and appear infected. Pruritus is variable and can be absent.

Fig. 5.7 Nummular dermatitis.

Diagnosis

Classic nummular dermatitis is generally easy to diagnose, but atypical cases may resemble a primary infective problem, psoriasis, or allergic contact dermatitis. The distribution of the lesions, generally sparing the knees, elbows, and scalp, is unlike psoriasis. Patch testing will identify most patients with allergic contact dermatitis, a few of whom, particularly women with nickel dermatitis and hand lesions, have a nummular pattern of dermatitis.

Treatment

Topical corticosteroids are the most effective means of controlling this condition. As secondary infection is common, the use of a steroid–antibiotic combination (for example betamethasone valerate + chinoform (Betnovate C)) is logical and may clear the lesions. In more persistent cases the application of 0.5–2 per cent tar or ichthyol in zinc paste will be beneficial. Systemic antipruritics are rarely required.

Asteatotic eczema (eczema craquelé)

This term is used to describe the dry irritable skin seen mainly on the limbs of elderly patients. The skin is dry and has large scales with a 'crazy-paving' appearance (Fig. 5.8). It appears to be the result of loss of epidermal lubrication together, in many cases, with inadequately removed soap after a bed bath. The problem is extremely common in communities of elderly people.

Treatment

This consists of replacing the missing lubrication. Soap should be withdrawn and emulsifying ointment BP, Ung. Merck, Moisturel, or a similar preparation used. Adequate lubrication may require very regular application of emollients and a reduction in bathing. Topical steroids should be avoided as the underlying skin is already thin and fragile.

Fig. 5.8 Eczema craquele. Note redness and scaling on shin area.

Seborrhoeic dermatitis

Definition

Seborrhoeic dermatitis is seen in two distinct subsets of patients. The infantile form is characterized by large yellowish scales mainly on the scalp, face, and napkin area, and is usually self limiting. The adult form affects the face, scalp, and anterior chest, and is associated with apparent itch out of proportion to the relatively mild degree of scaling and erythema seen.

Prevalence and aetiology

Infantile seborrhoeic dermatitis is a relatively common condition in young babies, and may cause confusion with infantile atopic dermatitis. The aetiology is unknown. There does not appear to be any link between the infantile and

Fig. 5.9 Infantile seborrhoeic dermatitis. Severe scalp involvement with large yellow adherent scales.

Fig. 5.10 Infantile seborrhoeic dermatitis. Erythema and scaling are present, but there is no apparent pruritus.

Fig. 5.11 Seborrhoeic dermatitis. Note erythema, and scaling.

adult forms of seborrhoeic dermatitis, and there is no evidence that children who have seborrhoeic dermatitis as infants are at greater risk of adult dermatitis in their later lives.

Adult seborrhoeic dermatitis is less common but much more persistent. It appears to be most often seen in adult males and is often associated on the trunk with involvement of the hair follicles. This is called seborrhoeic folliculitis. A mild degree of seborrhoeic dermatitis is common among adults. In spite of the name, neither qualitative nor quantitative changes in sebaceous secretion have been found in either the infantile or the adult form. *Pityrosporum ovale* has been found in greater numbers than on normal skin in patients with seborrhoeic dermatitis, and a proportion of patients respond to topical antifungal therapy. These facts clearly incriminate *P. ovale* as an aetiological agent, although it is not yet established whether this is in a primary or a secondary role.

Clinical features

In infants the child usually presents in early infancy with large yellow scales on the scalp extending down onto the forehead (Fig. 5.9). The child usually also has involvement on the trunk (Fig. 5.10) napkin area, and the axillae. There does not appear to be any pruritus, as the child is usually eating and sleeping well. This is a valuable diagnostic point in favour of seborrhoeic dermatitis and against atopic dermatitis.

In adults, the eruption consists of discrete, asymptomatic or mildly pruritic, red to yellow, glazed-looking lesions, mainly on the trunk. The presternal area, the axillae, submammary folds, groins, and external ear are common sites. Facial lesions are commoner in men and may be very persistent (Fig. 5.11), particularly in the nasolabial fold. Lesions on the trunk (Fig. 5.12) may be circular, pale pink, and at times difficult to see despite symptoms.

The scalp is frequently involved, and the presenting complaint may be of severe and persistent dandruff (pityriasis capitis, seen as scaling and erythema on

Fig. 5.12 Seborrhoeic dermatitis involving the trunk of an adult patient.

the scalp). Eyebrow and eyelid involvement is common with early morning stickiness of the eyelids. This blepharitis can be very unresponsive to therapy. Overall, seborrhoeic dermatitis tends to be chronic with seasonal variations peculiar to the individual. Severe and persistent seborrhoeic dermatitis is seen in a high proportion of patients who are HIV positive (see p. 141).

Diagnosis

Confusion may arise with allergic contact dermatitis, psoriasis, and pityriasis versicolor. Patch testing will generally exclude a true contact allergy, and the greasy yellow appearance of the lesions and their distribution are pointers against psoriasis, but this may easily be confused, particularly when there are only scalp lesions present. In psoriasis, however, the lesions are easily palpable and well delineated with large coarse silvery scales, whereas in seborrhoeic dermatitis they are more diffuse with finer smaller scales. Mycological examination of scrapings from individual lesions will exclude pityriasis versicolor, and may show the presence of large numbers of the yeast, *P. ovale*.

Seborrhoeic folliculitis is often associated with seborrhoeic dermatitis of the trunk. This consists of multiple small papules based on the follicles, and is thought to be due to excessive colonization of the follicles by *P. versicolor* (Fig. 5.13). It can be very resistant to treatment.

Treatment

Seborrhoeic dermatitis is a chronic problem which tends to recur whatever treatment is chosen. At present, the treatment of choice is a topical imidazole antifungal such as ketoconazole cream and shampoo (Nizoral) UK and USA, sulconazole (Exelderm), UK; miconazole (Daktarin), UK; clotrimazole (Lotrimin), USA; econazole (Spectazole), USA. Oral imidazoles are effective but should only be considered if topical measure fail, and should not be used continuously on a long-term basis.

Fig. 5.13 Seborrhoeic folliculitis. The lesions are often minimal relative to the degree of discomfort.

The associated problem of seborrhoeic folliculitis is particularly difficult to treat, and may only respond to systemic imidazoles.

Weak potency topical steroids are also of value (for example 1 per cent hydrocortisone cream to face and flexures) but, as with imidazoles, the condition tends to recur.

Key Points

> Contact dermatitis may be caused by a direct irritant or by allergic contact.

Contact dermatitis

Contact dermatitis comprises two quite distinct problems. These are:

1. caused by a **direct irritant** action of a substance on the skin;

2. **allergic contact dermatitis** which occurs only in patients whose skin has previously been sensitized by a contact with an allergen. Fresh contact with the antigen elicits a dermatitis reaction mediated by specifically sensitized T lymphocytes. The role of the epidermal Langerhans cells in presenting the allergen and in making subsequent contact with T lymphocytes either in the skin or local lymph nodes is currently the subject of active investigation.

Some of the differences between direct irritant contact dermatitis and allergic contact dermatitis are shown in Table 5.3. Current figures suggest that in the UK direct irritant dermatitis is a much commoner problem than the allergic contact variety.

Direct irritant contact dermatitis

Definition

Dermatitis caused by exposure to a substance which has a damaging effect on the normal barrier function of the epidermis.

Incidence and aetiology

Irritant contact dermatitis may be:

Table 5.3.

Differences between direct irritant and allergic contact dermatitis

	Direct irritant	Allergic contact
Prevalence	Very common	Much less common
Prior exposure to substance	Not required	Essential
Affected sites	Sites of direct contact with little extension	Sites of contact and distant sites
Susceptibility	Everyone susceptible	Only some patients susceptible
Other associated skin diseases	Atopy predisposes	Prolonged use of topical medicaments for chronic skin disease (e.g. leg ulcers) predisposes
Timing	Rapid onset 4–12 hours after contact. Lesions develop at first exposure	Onset generally 24 hours or longer after exposure. No lesions on first exposure

- **acute** due to a single exposure to an irritant substance;
- **subacute** due to repeated exposures of a small area as in napkin dermatitis;
- **chronic** 'wear and tear' due to repeated exposures to materials which deplete the normal protective film of lipid in and on the epidermis.

Acute irritant dermatitis is seen after one single, usually accidental, exposure to a strong skin irritant such as acid, alkali, phenol, halide, or quaternary ammonium compounds. The onset is rapid and lesions appear exactly at the sites of contact.

Subacute irritant dermatitis: here there is ongoing irritation as in infantile napkin dermatitis.

Chronic irritant dermatitis: a classic example of **cumulative exposure** to a mild cutaneous irritant is 'washerwoman's hands' due to continual contact with detergents and/or alkalis which degrease the skin and remove the protective lipid film. Chronic skin damage then develops.

Mild examples of cumulative insult irritant dermatitis are extremely common among persons regularly exposed to detergents and degreasing agents either at work or at home, and patients with atopic dermatitis are particularly susceptible. Many sufferers are convinced that they have an allergy, and may need a very clear explanation as to why this is not the problem.

Clinical features

After exposure to a strong irritant the affected skin becomes reddish-brown and vesicles develop. The lesions appear rapidly, usually within 6–12 hours of contact, and are painful and itchy. If there is no further contact with the irritant, recovery is rapid and it is unusual for lesions to develop at distant body sites. Identification of the aetiological agent depends on a careful history and, as the site and timing of the lesions are clear-cut, the patient himself will usually identify the substance in question.

In subacute dermatitis waves of fresh exposure confuse the clinical and pathological picture. There is erythema with crusting and sometimes blistering. There may also be early acanthosis and skin thickening. In infantile seborrhoeic dermatitis, (Fig. 5.14) the child has extensive erythema, sometimes with erosions and blistering on the napkin area, with striking sparing of the skin folds which have been relatively protected from the direct irritant effect of urine and faeces. This is in contrast to napkin candidosis in which the occlusive environment of the skin folds encourages candida overgrowth.

Chronic irritant dermatitis tends, initially, to present as dry, hacked, or fissured areas of skin which are susceptible to secondary infection. This is seen typically in housewives and young mothers whose hands are repeatedly exposed to soap, detergents, and water (Fig. 5.15). These substances tend to accumulate under rings and, with the added effect of local trauma, may provoke severe reactions which are clinically very similar to those seen as a result of allergic contact sensitivity to metals. Patch testing may be needed to rule out allergic contact dermatitis.

Fig. 5.14 Napkin dermatitis. Severe involvement with relative sparing of skin flexures.

Fig. 5.15 Chronic wear and tear dermatitis on the backs of the hands.

Treatment

Identification of the irritant and its subsequent avoidance is the cornerstone of successful therapy. The cause is identified on the patient's history. Patch testing to standard allergens may be needed to rule out allergic contact dermatitis.

For the active phase, a topical steroid cream or ointment is usually the most appropriate treatment. If the lesions are acute with vesicles and weeping, wet dressings applied as soaks or lotions may be needed until the subacute phase is reached, when topical steroids can be substituted. Suitable wet dressings and lotions include aluminium acetate lotion 5 per cent in sterile water, and calamine lotion BP (15 per cent calamine, 5 per cent zinc oxide, and 5 per cent glycerine). Prior soaking of the area in a weak solution of 0.01–0.1 per cent potassium permanganate in water for 5 minutes may be soothing and help to prevent secondary infection. The choice of topical steroid for the subacute phase is wide and, as the surface area involved may be small and the condition of short duration, the use of a relatively strong steroid is justified. Suitable examples are 0.1 per cent betamethasone 17-valerate with 3 per cent clioquinol in a water miscible base (Betnovate C), fluocinolone acetonide (Synalar), or beclomethasone dipropionate 0.025 per cent (Propaderm). As acute reactions seldom become chronic, keratolytics are rarely indicated.

Children with napkin dermatitis should have all napkins removed and be nursed in a warm dry environment with the skin exposed. Lesions will rapidly resolve if this is done and improvement will be accelerated by the use of a mild steroid antifungal combination such as miconazole/hydrocortisone (Daktacort). The mother should, however, be warned that this should not become the child's regular napkin cream, and topical steroids should be withdrawn when the skin returns to normal.

The management of chronic cumulative irritant contact dermatitis is protection of the area involved, most commonly the hands, from exposure to the cause and the liberal use of emollients to replace the lipid barrier. Patients should be warned that up to 6 months daily application of emollients may be needed before the skin regains its barrier function and former resilience.

Prevention of irritant dermatitis is theoretically simple. All individual workers at risk should be issued with appropriate advice, barrier creams, and protective clothing. Chronic detergent contact with hands should be prevented by using occlusive vinyl (not rubber) gloves and underneath these a thin pair of cotton gloves to absorb perspiration. This is much more effective than flock or cotton-lined gloves. Thorough rinsing of the hands after essential soap and water exposure is important as is the regular use of emollient preparations to hydrate the skin (for example emulsifying ointment BP, Ung. Merck). Routine use of topical steroids for this purpose is not appropriate.

Allergic contact dermatitis

Definition

Dermatitis caused by prior exposure to an allergen leading to specific cell-mediated sensitization.

Prevalence and aetiology

This form of dermatitis affects 1–2 per cent of the population. Certain groups are at greater risk. Patients with chronic skin conditions, such as leg ulcers, tend to become sensitized to medicaments, and workers exposed to common sensitizers, such as chromates in the building industry or dyes and tanning agents in leather manufacture, have a higher incidence than the population at large.

The commonest sensitizing agents in Europe and North America have been identified, and they can be used as a standard or routine battery of around 20 patch tests for investigating patients with this type of dermatitis. Substances in this battery are changed as appropriate according to observed changes in clinical problems, but include nickel and chromates, rubber breakdown products, preservatives, topical antibiotics, and topical steroid molecules. The current European battery is listed in Table 5.4. In addition, smaller groups of relevant allergens are used when investigating specific problems, for example a 'footwear battery' for chronic foot dermatitis, a medicament battery for leg ulcers, and a cosmetic battery for facial problems.

In theory, once the offending allergen has been identified by patch testing, and thereafter avoided, rapid clearance of the skin lesions should occur, but in practice this is not always the case. Certain common allergens are very difficult to avoid in the course of everyday life and nickel is a good example. It is found in cutlery, coins, cooking implements, gardening and motoring equipment, jewellery, household furniture, and many other items, and it can be extremely difficult, even for an intelligent and motivated patient, to avoid nickel contact. There is evidence that even trace amounts of nickel in the diet may play a part in perpetuating the skin lesions.

Table 5.4.

Materials currently used in the European Standard Battery for patch testing.

0.5% potassium dichromate	20% neomycin sulphate
1% thiuram mix	1% paraphenylene diamine base
1% cobalt chloride	5% benzocaine
1% formaldehyde	20% colophony
6% quinolone mix	25% balsam of Peru
0.6% PPD black rubber mix	30% wool alcohols
2% mercapto mix	15% epoxy resin
15% paraben mix	1% BPP resin
1% ethylenediaminedihydrochloride	1% Dowicil 200
5% nickel sulphate	0.1% kathon
2% mercaptobenzothiazole	8% fragrance mix
1% tixocortol pivalate	0.1% primin
0.1% budesonide	

The medico-legal consequences of allergic contact dermatitis acquired through exposure to allergens at work are considerable. Contact dermatitis is classified as an industrial injury, in the UK and some other countries patients are entitled to financial compensation. Prevention by removing the sufferer from the allergen containing environment or by removing the allergen from the process for which the patient is responsible is theoretically possible, but clearly requires collaboration between the work-force, industrial medical officers, and others.

Clinical features

Allergic contact dermatitis usually presents with acute or subacute dermatitis lesions at sites where the allergen is, or has been, in direct contact with the skin and also with milder involvement of more distant areas where there has been no obvious direct contact. As sensitization may develop after many years of trouble-free daily contact with the allergen, the patient may be unaware that he is reacting to this particular substance and even after positive patch testing it may be very hard to convince him that a material handled regularly for many years is now to be avoided.

Common sites of involvement are the ear lobes and nape of neck (nickel in jewellery, Fig. 5.16 and 5.17), the wrist (metal or leather watch straps or bracelets), and the feet (tanning agents used in curing leather, adhesives used for fixing insoles, dyes used for leather or socks, glue used in assembling shoes,

Fig. 5.16 (*above right*) Nickel dermatitis showing striking reaction to nickel coin.

Fig. 5.17 (*above*) Same patient showing striking reaction on conventional patch testing to both nickel and cobalt.

Fig. 5.18 Shoe dermatitis. After topical treatment patch tests were performed and a positive result obtained to potassium dichromate.

Fig. 5.18). A problem recognized relatively recently is that of sensitization to the corticosteroid molecule. This should always be considered when a patient has dermatitis which appears to deteriorate while on steroid therapy.

In the early stages the affected area is inflamed and itchy, with papules and vesicles. Continued exposure to the allergen will lead to dryness, scaling, and fissuring. This picture may be complicated when renewed exposure causes an acute or subacute exacerbation to develop on the background of a long-standing chronic dermatitis. The lesions frequently spread well beyond the area of contact with the allergen and also even to distant body sites which have not been in contact with the allergen. The main site of involvement may give a useful clue to the cause and Table 5.5 lists such common sites and likely agents. Exposure to sensitizing plants, particularly to primula, tends to cause a blistering eruption

Table 5.5.

Principal sites of allergic contact dermatitis and likely causes

Site	Likely cause
Face	Cosmetics, perfume in toilet soap, nickel, plastic spectacle frames, medicaments (e.g. antibiotics in eye or ear drops) (Fig. 5.19)
Scalp	Hair dyes (paraphenylenediamine—PPD), lotions and tonics containing Balsam of Peru
Mouth	Denture materials
Neck and ear lobes	Nickel containing jewellery
Wrists	Nickel, PPD, chromates–jewellery and leather watch straps
Hands	Plants (e.g. primulas), nickel (begins under rings), material handled in occupation or recreation, lanolin (hand creams, medicaments)
Body	Nickel jeanstuds or rubber material in underwear, clothing dyes
Feet	Dyes used in socks and shoes glues, chromates, etc. in shoes

relatively rapidly on the sites of actual contact and also a general facial erythema due to airborne allergen.

Hand dermatitis tends to be a common and persistent problem in individuals sensitive to nickel. In all cases of persistent hand dermatitis it is good practice both to patch test to exclude an avoidable allergen and to examine scrapings for fungi to exclude a fungal infection.

Treatment

The management of allergic contact dermatitis is divided logically into four stages.

1. **Detection of the likely sensitizing agent** by taking a careful occupational, recreational, and medicament history. Knowledge of the common sensitizers and the sites they may affect is obviously necessary at this stage.
2. **Preparation for valid patch testing** to identify the allergen. It is essential to avoid all materials thought to be possibly responsible for the eruption while applying a topical steroid preparation to clear the dermatitis. The presence of active lesions even at distant body sites while patch testing is carried out will result in both false positive and false negative results, and all lesions must therefore be cleared *before* patch tests are performed.

Fig. 5.19 Medicament dermatitis. This patient had recently received an eye ointment containing neomycin.

Topical steroid preparations are helpful. The strength of steroid used should be chosen according to the site involved—facial lesions should receive a mild preparation (for example clobetasone butyrate, Eumovate) while the thicker skin of the hands and feet require a stronger preparation (for example fluocinolone acetonide, Synalar). Most centres prefer to avoid patch testing until the skin has been relatively free of inflammation for 4–6 weeks, and the area to which the patches are to be applied has not been treated with topical steroids for 1–2 weeks but this is not always possible. Pregnancy has an effect on the immune system and thus on the results of patch testing so if possible it is best to delay patch testing until after delivery to obtain a relevant result.

3. **Patch testing** to the suspected substances (for the technique, see p. 41). In practice it is common to test patients with all substances in the European standard battery plus any other likely allergens, for example small pieces cut from the inner aspects of shoes in foot dermatitis. This can be done using chemicals stored in syringes and applied to inert metal chambers, or by using prepared strips of patches (Trutest). The patches are left in position for 48 hours, removed, and the area examined for redness and swelling at that time and also 48 hours later. Patch test results can be surprisingly difficult to interpret, as some allergens are also irritants and irritant reactions can, to the non-expert, look very like a true positive result.

4. **Counselling on avoidance of responsible allergens** following patch test results. This is not always straightforward. For example, although it may be easy to avoid the plant in primula dermatitis, it is much more difficult to obtain appropriate allergen free footwear in shoe dermatitis. There are difficulties in industry when a skilled worker finds it hard to avoid exposure to an allergen, and factory or industrial medical officers may be of great assistance in such cases.

It is essential that these four stages of treatment and investigation be followed. A delay in response to treatment prior to patch testing (stage 2) may be due to continuing exposure to the aetiological agent. This is particularly common in medicament-induced contact dermatitis and in such cases topical preparations containing lanolin or preservatives (for example parabens) should be avoided. The possibility of topical corticosteroid sensitivity should also be considered.

Dishydrotic eczema (pompholyx)

This term is used to describe a very characteristic pattern of intensely itchy vesicles of the skin of the hands—cheiropompholyx—and occasionally also the feet—cheiropodopompholyx. The sides of the finger are frequently involved and clinically the individual lesions have a 'sago grain' or 'frog spawn' appearance due to translucent deeply-set papules (Fig. 5.20). These are often easier to feel than to see.

The cause of this pattern of dermatitis is not understood. In some cases patients have allergic contact dermatitis, especially to nickel. In other cases no specific allergen is found, but the problem appears to be aggravated by stress.

Key Points

In chronic persistent hand dermatitis, arrange for patch tests to identify unexpected allergens. Eighty per cent of all contact dermatitis involves the hands and forearms.

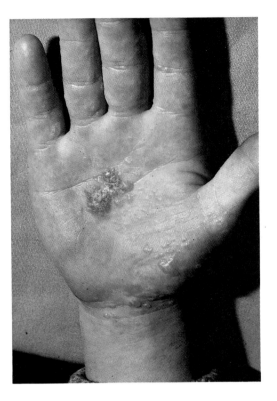

Fig. 5.20 Cheiropompholyx involving the palms and side of the fingers.

Treatment

Systemic antihistamines will help control the need to scratch and thus prevent secondary infection. The intense, but usually short-lived, itch is best treated for a short time with potent topical steroids. If the lesions are very moist, wet soaks, using calamine lotion may be helpful.

Neurodermatitis (circumscribed lichen simplex)

Definition

A well-demarcated area of chronic lichenified dermatitis which is not due to either external irritants or identified allergens.

Aetiology

In predisposed persons the lesions are induced by continual scratching or rubbing of a localized area of itchy skin. The initial pruritic stimulus, which seems to be related to stress or emotional disturbance, generates an itch-scratch-itch cycle. This, in turn, stimulates a reactive epidermal hyperplasia recognized clinically as lichenification (Fig. 5.21).

Fig. 5.21 Neurodermatitis showing dark thickened area over skin of right scapula.

Neurodermatitis is relatively uncommon and the diagnosis should be made after excluding commoner causes of dermatitis, for example irritant or allergic contact dermatitis. It is commoner in women than in men.

Clinical features

Usually the isolated, well-circumscribed, lichenified, slightly elevated plaques are seen on the nape of the neck, the forearms, or the legs. They have a characteristic mauve colour and accentuation of normal skin markings. Affected patients are often tense and obsessive, and there appears to be an association with atopy.

Diagnosis and treatment

A biopsy may occasionally be necessary to confirm the diagnosis when individual lesions resemble psoriasis or even lichen planus. An atypical fungal infection could also cause confusion. Mycological examination will exclude this possibility.

Treatment should be aimed at breaking the itch-scratch-itch cycle and consists of antihistamines by mouth to reduce pruritus, topical corticosteroids to suppress inflammation, and tar or ichthyol-containing preparations for their antipruritic and keratolytic effects. Occlusive dressings prevent scratching and are the most effective treatment. For lesions on a limb, a tar or ichthyol impregnated bandage (for example Coltapaste, Ichthopaste) applied for a week may totally clear the lesion. Unfortunately, however, recurrence after removal of occlusion is frequent. In some cases intralesional injections of a steroid preparation such as triamcinolone may be beneficial.

Prurigo nodularis

This problem can be regarded as a variant of neurodermatitis. As a result of itch and subsequent scratching, lichenified nodules develop. They may be as large as 1–5 cm in diameter, and the clinical differential diagnosis may include skin tumours. The history of chronic severe itch is helpful, but a biopsy may be necessary to establish the diagnosis. Potent topical steroids under occlusive dressings are the most useful form of treatment.

Stasis dermatitis

Definition

An area of dermatitis on the lower legs, commonly seen in association with venous insufficiency or frank ulceration.

Incidence and aetiology

A large number of obese, usually female, patients have a degree of venous insufficiency or frank varicose veins of the lower limbs. Prior to the development of frank stasis ulcers (p. 174) a mild dermatitis reaction associated with epidermal atrophy, purpura, and pigmentation due to haemosiderin may develop. These changes are related to extravasation of blood into the tissues and poor oxygenation.

Clinical features

The inner aspects of both lower legs above and around the medial malleolus are chiefly involved. The skin is shiney, atrophic, and usually has large numbers of small blood vessels clearly visible (Fig. 5.22). Pruritus may be severe and cause scratch marks which are slow to heal. Other less severe lesions may be seen on the calves and thighs.

Fig. 5.22 Varicose eczema showing atrophy and tissue breakdown around the malleolus.

Treatment

Treatment of underlying varicose veins is the most important form of therapy. The use of topical steroids, although symptomatically valuable, is not recommended long-term as it will accelerate the atrophic changes in what is already thin epidermis. Protective ichthyol or tar-impregnated bandages are useful both in preventing scratching and in protecting from other forms of minor trauma.

Patient association

The National Eczema Society is a patient support group with branches in many countries which offer support and practical advice to sufferers from all types of dermatitis and eczema, although a high proportion of members have atopic dermatitis. The Society produces a number of well-researched and medically approved information packs.

Discussion of problem cases (see p. 77)

Case 5.1

The history is strongly suggestive of atopic dermatitis. The mother gives a history of seasonal rhinitis, so the child has an atopic background. No laboratory tests are necessary to confirm the diagnosis. The parents needed time and a careful explanation of the nature of atopic dermatitis, including the fact that it is usually self limiting. Printed leaflets will help enforce verbal explanations. The child was carefully examined to exclude the possibility of secondary problems, particularly eczema herpeticum. Emollients and a soap substitute were prescribed, and the mother asked to avoid woollen clothing next the baby's skin, substituting cotton. One per cent hydrocortisone ointment was prescribed as the initial steroid, and oral promethazine for night time sedation. A dermatology nurse spent time with the parents showing them how to apply dressings. The parents were given the address of the National Eczema Society.

The mother returned 2 weeks later with the child who was much improved but still scratching and rubbing his legs. A moderate potency steroid was prescribed for this area, and one month later his skin was itchy but looked relatively normal. He continued to require prescriptions for hydrocortisone and night sedation for the next 9 months, and his skin flared with episodes of teething and minor coughs and colds. By the age of 2 years his skin was dry but non-inflamed and apparently non-pruritic.

The parents ask you about the likelihood of any further children being affected. How would you reply?

Case 5.2

This presentation tends to be a bit of a heartsink case for a dermatologist. The history and presentation strongly suggest seborrhoeic dermatitis and associated seborrhoeic folliculitis. Both are very difficult to clear completely. The pattern of involvement on the face and scalp with sparing of the fingers does not suggest scabies.

The patient was given topical imidazole (ketoconazole) cream and shampoo, and this improved the problems on his face and scalp but did not affect the itch on his trunk. At his request and, after discussion, he was given a 4 week course of oral imidazole (fluconazole) with again little benefit. This was stopped, and he had a six week course of UVB therapy, but was concerned about future skin cancer risks so this also was stopped, and he was given simple 2 per cent menthol in calamine cream with a little symptomatic relief. At the next visit, he tells you he is emigrating to the US.

Are there any other treatment options to consider here?

Case 5.3

Young individuals embarking on a hairdressing career often have hand dermatitis problems, particularly in the first year when they are working as juniors, and spend a lot of time shampooing—thus in contact with water and detergent. Most salons will not let them wear latex or rubber gloves, so the cumulative drying effect to the skin is considerable.

This is the most likely explanation in this case. Patch testing was carried out to exclude an allergic cause, and as expected the results were negative, although difficult to interpret because of some irritant reactions.

She was advised to use copious amounts of emollients, and to wear cotton under rubber gloves as much as possible. Her skin slowly improved on this routine, and she was able to continue to train as a hairdresser.

Case 5.4

The patient has visible varicose veins and the history suggests associated stasis dermatitis. Once the dermatitis has been treated she should be referred for consideration for surgical treatment of her varicose veins. The preparation she was using on her leg was a lanolin containing steroid cream, not a recommended therapy for stasis dermatitis because of the skin thinning effect of topical steroids. However, in the short-term they should not actually aggravate pre-existing dermatitis.

Because of this history, the patients was patch tested and was found to be sensitive to lanolin. Her leg was treated with ichthopaste bandages, and when the dermatitis had settled her varicose veins were surgically treated. Three months later the skin around her ankles was relatively normal.

What advice do you give her about her lanolin allergy?

Projects

1. Run a literature search on genes causing atopy. Review as many of the papers as you can. How many of them report on respiratory atopy, how many on cutaneous atopy, and how many on the two combined? What are the results from these three subsets? What conclusions can you draw from this overview?

2. You are asked by the head teacher of a local primary school (children aged 5–11) to prepare an information sheet for teachers about atopic dermatitis so that they can give support to the children in the school with the problem. Write this using no more than 1000 words. How could you audit the value of this information sheet?

Growth points

1. **Latex allergy**

There is currently considerable concern about type 1 hypersensitivity to latex caused by the use of latex gloves. This is particularly prevalent in hospital workers, and can cause dramatic and severe respiratory problems. It is also a potential hazard for patients as catheters and endotracheal tubes contain latex. The problem can be partly avoided by the use of vinyl gloves, and by using good quality rubber gloves from a reliable source with low levels of extractable latex.

2. **Topical corticosteroid allergy**

Current UK figures suggest that 6 per cent of those referred for contact dermatitis investigation are sensitive to one or more topical steroids. Budesonide and tixocortol pivalate are the two which appear to cause sensitization most commonly in relation to the quantities prescribed. When patch testing for steroid allergy it is important to use the steroid in an alcohol base, as the traditional test carried out using a petrolatum or cream base may give false negative results.

Further reading

Fisher, A.A. (1995). *Contact dermatitis*, (4th edn). Lea and Feibiger, Philadelphia.

Ruzicka, T., Ring, J., and Przybilla, B. (ed.) (1991) *Handbook of atopic dermatitis.* Springer Verlag, Berlin.

Rycroft, R.J.G., Menne, T., and Frosch, P. (1995) *Textbook of contact dermatitis,* (2nd edn). Springer Verlag, Berlin.

6

Cutaneous infections and infestations

- **Bacterial infections:**   Impetigo
                               Erysipelas
                               Cellulitis
                               Erythrasma
- **Mycobacterial:**   Tuberculosis
                               Leprosy
- **Viral:**   Warts
                               Molluscum contagiosum
                               Orf
                               Herpes simplex
                               Herpes zoster
- **Spirochaetal:**   Lyme disease
- **Fungal:**   Candida
                               Dermatophyte infections
                               Pityriasis versicolor
- **Protozoal:**   Leishmaniasis
- **Infestations:**   Scabies
                               Pediculosis capitis
                               Pediculosis corporis
                               Pediculosis pubis
- **Sexually transmitted disease:** Syphilis
                               Gonorrhoea
                               Reiter's disease
- **Dermatological complications of HIV infection:**
                               Kaposi's sarcoma
                               Hairy oral leukoplakia
                               Severe candidosis
                               Severe herpes simplex
                               Severe seborrhoeic dermatitis
                               Deterioration of psoriasis

Problem cases

Case 6.1

A 7-year-old boy is brought to you by his mother. He has a history of atopic dermatitis, which still troubles him in the winter months, mainly on his face and in the popliteal fossae. In the past 3 days he has developed widespread but superficial crusting on his cheeks. He is otherwise well.

What is the differential diagnosis here, what investigations might be useful and what therapy would you prescribe?

Case 6.2

A 43-year-old farmer's wife comes to your clinic with a scaling lesion at the top of her left thigh. Her family doctor in his letter calls this an isolated patch of psoriasis, and initially you prescribe calcipotriol. She returns one month later and there is no change. On closer inspection you see that the centre of the plaque is atrophic and scarred, and that the edge of the lesion does not have the classic scaling of psoriasis. The patient is quite definite that the mark, which she considers a birthmark, has been there for 40 years.

What might your clinical differential diagnosis be and what investigations would be useful?

Case 6.3

A young Asian couple bring their 2-year-old daughter to see you because of loss of normal pigmentation on her right forearm. The child is otherwise well, but the parents are clearly very concerned. The child was born in Pakistan and only came to the UK 3 months ago.

What are the causes of painless loss of normal pigmentation, and how would you establish a diagnosis?

Case 6.4

You are consulted by the mother of an 18-year-old girl, who is on dialysis and awaiting a kidney transplant, about an unrelated matter. In passing, she mentions that her daughter has both hand and genital warts. The mother wants to know if she should be treated now, or wait until after the transplant when she will feel fitter.

What is the best approach in this case?

Case 6.5

A 38-year-old college lecturer consults you about a red, painful right calf. He has just returned from a weekend walking in the New Forest area of the UK, and wonders if he has an allergy to his new walking boots.

Discuss the possible differential diagnosis, the appropriate investigations, and the suggested treatment.

Case 6.6

You are asked to visit a retirement home because several of the old ladies in the home have developed itchy skin lesions. Five elderly ladies who share a room all have scaling and itch involving most of the trunk and limbs, and you are told that a nurse who has just gone on holiday has the same problem. Before you have seen the patients topical hydrocortisone has been applied to the affected areas with very little benefit. The senior nurse in charge is concerned about a change in the detergent used for laundry.

What are the possible causes of this outbreak, what investigations might be helpful, and what treatments would be appropriate?

In Britain, Europe, and North America the problem of bacterial cutaneous infection has fallen over the past two decades. It is still important, however, to be able to recognize and treat these conditions promptly. Unfortunately, there has been no such decline in the incidence of viral or fungal cutaneous infections, and recent advances in therapy has made it possible to treat previously intractable problems. Cutaneous infestation continues to be a problem of poor hygiene and overcrowding, and there is currently a rising incidence of various forms of sexually transmitted disease. HIV related problems including atypical and resistant forms of tuberculosis and other infections are becoming commoner, and must be recognized. All of these will be discussed in this chapter.

Bacterial Infections

Impetigo

Definition

A superficial cutaneous infection caused by either staphylococci or streptococci.

Incidence and aetiology

Impetigo is easily spread in situations such as day nurseries where there is frequent contact between children.

The organisms commonly identified in impetigo are *Staphylococcus aureus* and group A streptococci. The disease is much commoner in children, and can present as a very thin-roofed, quickly ruptured blister, especially when caused by staphylococci.

Key Points

Impetigo (a superficial infection by staphylococci or streptococci) usually responds quickly to topical antibiotic but systemic antibiotics are required to prevent post-streptococcal glomerulonephritis.

Clinical features

The hallmark of impetigo is a superficial lesion covered with a heavy honey-coloured crust, usually on the face and hands. Impetigo can develop very rapidly and may complicate a pre-existing skin condition such as atopic dermatitis or acne (Fig. 6.1).

Management

Removal of crusts with warm saline or olive oil soaks and the application of a topical antibiotic, such as aureomycin, fucidin, or mupirocin (Bactroban), are the essential points in management. The infection in impetigo is extremely superficial and therefore most cases will respond quickly and heal with no scarring.

While the use of systemic antibiotics in impetigo is only essential if streptococci have been shown to be present, as the aim is to prevent post-streptococcal glomerulonephritis, it is common practice in the majority of severe cases also to prescribe full doses of oral penicillin or erythromycin for 5–7 days.

Erysipelas

Definition

A cutaneous streptococcal infection characterized by sharply demarcated unilateral lesions, commonly on the face.

Clinical features

Erysipelas presents as a bright red, brawny, oedematous area. The face is most frequently affected. The organism gains entry through a minor abrasion and infects the superficial lymphatic vessels. The lesions are unilateral, and associated with leucocytosis and fever (Fig. 6.2).

Diagnosis and treatment

Prompt response to full doses of oral penicillin is the most useful diagnostic test for erysipelas. Although swabs should be taken routinely for bacteriological confirmation, the results should not be awaited before starting therapy. Topical therapy is unnecessary, but many dermatologists routinely prescribe a topical antibiotic. Topical steroids should be withheld, as they will delay response to systemic antibiotic therapy.

In a proportion of cases recurrent erysipelas develops on the same site, leading in time to chronic lymphoedema. Management of this complication is difficult and, although long-term antibiotic therapy is used, results are not always satisfactory.

Cellulitis

Definition

A cutaneous infection, usually due to streptococci, but with deeper involvement of the subcutis than in erysipelas.

Fig. 6.1 Staphylococcal impetigo superimposed on mild atopic dermatitis. Note gross honey-coloured crusting.

Fig. 6.2 Erysipelas. Note well-demarcated edge to the lesion. Response to oral penicillin within 24 hours is normal.

Fig. 6.3 Cellulitis involving the skin of the lower leg and ankle. Note intense swelling and erythema.

Clinical features

Cellulitis presents as a raised, hot, tender, erythematous area of skin (Fig. 6.3). The organism enters through a cut or abrasion, or a pre-existing dermatological disorder such as a leg ulcer. The affected area is larger and more diffuse than in erysipelas and the edges are not so well demarcated. Fever and leucocytosis are common. The draining lymph nodes are usually palpable and tender.

Diagnosis and treatment

Diagnosis is usually straightforward and therapy should be commenced immediately with full doses of a systemic antibiotic. Bacteriological swabs should be taken to identify the causative organism and to test for its antibiotic sensitivity. When these results are available the antibiotic can, if necessary, be changed. The initial choice of antibiotic will depend on the patient and his environment. In an otherwise healthy young person seen outside hospital streptococcus is likely to be the cause and full doses of penicillin V are appropriate. On the other hand, in the elderly or in patients who have impaired immunity, a variety of organisms may be responsible and a broad-spectrum antibiotic (for example flucloxacillin) should be used. Blood cultures should be taken before starting therapy in this situation.

Erythrasma

Definition

A cutaneous infection caused by *Corynebacterium minutissimum.*

Clinical features

Erythrasma causes an asymptomatic, reddish-brown area of skin, commonly in body flexures, particularly the groin. It does not appear to be contagious and, if untreated, it spreads slowly with a well-demarcated advancing edge.

Diagnosis and treatment

Erythrasma can be diagnosed both by bacteriological identification of *Corynebacterium minutissimum* and by the coral-red fluorescence seen under Wood's light. Clinical confusion with a superficial fungal infection is resolved by these procedures.

Topical imidazoles such as clotrimazole or miconazole, or topical erythromycin are all effective. Full doses of erythromycin by mouth (250 mg four times per day for 7 days) are also curative but rarely needed.

Mycobacterial Infection

Tuberculosis

Although 'classical' tuberculosis is now uncommon in Britain, it must still be remembered and promptly treated in the elderly, in the immunosuppressed, and in immigrant populations with less natural resistance to *Mycobacterium tuberculosis*. In many parts of the world there is at present an upsurge of tuberculosis infection in immunosuppressed individuals, and in many cases there appears to be resistance to classic antituberculous drugs. In this section of the population, tuberculosis can appear in atypical forms, and it is important always to consider tuberculosis in any stubborn and atypical skin problem in immunocompromised individuals.

Lupus vulgaris

Definition

The commonest form of cutaneous tuberculosis occurring after primary infection in individuals with good natural resistance to *M. tuberculosis*.

Incidence and aetiology

Lupus vulgaris (LV) is most common in northern Europe and affects females more often than males. Children are more frequently affected and in the elderly it may present with reactivation of old lesions following inadequate treatment in the past.

Pathology

Discrete, well-formed, tuberculoid granulomata are seen in the mid-dermis. Caseation is rare and the mycobacteria will only exceptionally be identified in Gram-stained sections, or by culture or guinea-pig inoculation.

Clinical features

Lupus vulgaris most commonly affects the face and neck and is seen initially as firm, translucent, brown nodules (Fig. 6.4). These are called 'apple jelly nodules' because of their appearance on diascopy. This is gentle pressure on the lesion with a transparent glass slide or coverslip to impede local blood flow.

Key Points

Classic tuberculosis is uncommon in Britain but may be present in some populations (the elderly, the immunosuppressed, and some immigrants) where its appearance may be atypical and carry resistance.

Fig. 6.4 Lupus vulgaris. Note yellow-brown translucent tinge to lesion.

Fig. 6.5 Lupus vulgaris showing striking scarring and continuing activity on skin on right side of the neck.

Fig. 6.6 Scrofuloderma. Here *M. tuberculosis* can be cultured from the ulcerated area which is in direct contact with an infected lymph node underlying the ulcer.

Untreated, the lesions will slowly spread laterally, giving rise to disfiguring scarring and contractions (Fig. 6.5). Malignant change has been reported in these scars, even in patients who have not received therapeutic X-rays or large doses of UV light in the past.

Diagnosis and treatment

Biopsy and culture should be performed to confirm the diagnosis and then the patient should receive full antituberculous therapy for at least one year. Current practice is to give three antituberculous drugs. The current drugs of choice are rifampicin, isonicotinic acid hydrazide (INAH), and pyrazinamide. Ethambutol is used if resistance is suspected, and rifabutin is useful as prophylaxis in those with low CD4 counts.

Scrofuloderma

Definition

Cutaneous tuberculosis due to spread of the organisms via sinuses from underlying caseous lymph nodes.

Clinical features: an ulcerated area is seen usually on the neck, overlying palpable lymph nodes (Fig. 6.6). Recognition is easy as *M. tuberculosis* can be identified both in the nodes and in the material draining onto the skin surface.

Treatment: full antituberculous therapy is required. The recommended drugs are as for lupus vulgaris.

Leprosy (Hansen's Disease)

Air travel and the presence of a large immigrant population in parts of many countries make it important for both family doctors and dermatologists to recognize, or at least suspect, the commoner presentations of leprosy. Although the condition is rare in Europe and North America, undiagnosed cases of leprosy can spread infection amongst a wide range of contacts, particularly the young and the elderly.

The polar varieties of *Mycobacterium leprae* infection are tuberculoid and lepromatous, but in current practice, most patients have borderline or mixed infection. The tuberculoid form is associated with low infectivity and a high degree of natural resistance to the organism, whereas the lepromatous type is associated with large numbers of easily identified micro-organisms, a high degree of infectivity, and little natural resistance to the mycobacteria. In between these two extremes lies a range of presentations combining features of both polar forms. Borderline or dimorphous leprosy and indeterminate leprosy are terms used to describe these clinical problems.

Pathology

In tuberculoid leprosy well-formed granulomata invade the dermis from within the nerve trunks which are the primary site of infection. Cutaneous nerves may have been destroyed by this process and *M. leprae* will rarely be seen despite careful microscopy.

Fig. 6.7 Tuberculoid leprosy. Note obvious areas of depigmentation which were also anaesthetic.

In lepromatous leprosy the granulomata generally lie deeper in the dermis and contain a large proportion of foamy histiocytes (macrophages). *M. leprae* are presented in large numbers in these cells and can be easily identified with special stains (for example Ziehl–Nielsen).

Key Points

Do not forget leprosy as a cause of pigment loss in dark skinned individuals.

Clinical features

In tuberculoid leprosy the infection is mainly in the peripheral nerves and the cutaneous manifestation is likely to be an anaesthetic macule or plaque with pigmentary changes. On white skin this may show as an erythematous or brown discoloration, but on colored skin depigmentation is commonly seen. Palpable peripheral nerves may be felt near the area of discoloration. As skin appendages are damaged by the process, sweating and hair growth are diminished or absent. The lesions tend to develop adjacent to scars and vaccination sites, and they are sparse in the pure tuberculoid type (Fig. 6.7).

In borderline cases the lesions are similar but more numerous.

In lepromatous leprosy macules, papules, nodules, and ulceration develop at sites where tissue temperature is low, such as the nostrils which are frequently involved, leading to septal perforation, collapse of the nasal bones, and a characteristic deformity. Hair growth and sweating over the lesions is not impaired, and normal sensation is preserved. A generalized thickening of the involved facial tissues gives rise to a leonine facies, and severe and intractable leg ulcers may develop.

Diagnosis and treatment

The diagnosis should be confirmed and treatment started at a centre which has some experience of leprosy. A full-thickness skin biopsy, skin snips, a peripheral nerve biopsy, and the lepromin test are all diagnostic aids. The choice of which of these to use in individual cases depends on the clinical presentation.

Treatment is based on systemic sulphones, rifampicin, and clofazimine, although resistance is becoming a problem and in the initial stages it can be complicated by reactions, particularly in lepromatous leprosy. In the UK, there is a leprosy panel organized by the Department of Health who will give advice on best current therapy (phone number 0171 972 4480). The duration of treatment varies. The tuberculoid variety should be treated for 1–2 years after disease activity has ceased, but in the lepromatous variety treatment should continue for life. Children who are household contacts should be followed up as they can harbour the organism for many years and develop the disease in adult life. Adult contacts rarely become infected.

Viral Infections

Warts

Definition

Common benign cutaneous tumours caused by the human papilloma virus (HPV).

Warts are usually self-limiting cutaneous tumours caused by a range of DNA viruses, the human papilloma viruses (HPV). They vary significantly in their clinical presentation and different types of wart virus may be associated with specific clinical presentation (for example genital warts). The wart virus is transmitted by direct contact. A small number of the over 90 varieties of human papilloma virus currently recognised have oncogenic potential. This is of particular importance in immunosuppressed individuals such as organ transplant recipients.

Common wart (Verruca vulgaris)

These easily identified lesions are usually multiple, raised, hyperkeratotic, and are commonly found on the hands. They are particularly common in children aged 5–10 years and may be painful, especially when periungual. Common warts demonstrate the *Koebner phenomenon* (p. 33), and develop on sites of trauma.

Key Points

> Warts are self-limiting, benign tumours, caused by the human papilloma virus, that usually involute spontaneously.

Fig. 6.8 Multiple hand warts. Note extensive lesion on the dorsal of all fingers.

Fig. 6.9 Plane warts. Note the Koebner phenomenon caused by scratching.

Fig. 6.10 Multiple plantar warts. These can be both painful and difficult to treat.

All types of warts are more persistent in those whose cell-mediated immunity is suppressed. Renal transplant recipients, for example, tend to have large numbers of warts which stubbornly resist treatment (Fig. 6.8).

Plane warts

These occur most frequently on the face and the backs of hands. Each is a slightly raised circular or oval plaque. Despite their relatively banal appearance, they are surprisingly resistant to therapy (Fig. 6.9).

Plantar warts (Verruca plantaris)

Constant pressure and friction on the soles prevents the normal outward expansion of warts in this site, and instead they grow inwards towards the dermis (Fig. 6.10). Pressure on nerves can cause considerable pain. Children, sportsmen, athletes, and others who use communal showering facilities are particularly at risk.

Human papilloma viruses types 1 and 3 are the commonest types associated with cutaneous warts described above. They are not considered oncogenic varieties of HPV.

Genital warts

These warts tend to develop in large clusters. They affect the penile and vulvar skin, mucous membrane, and also the perianal area (Fig. 6.11). Sexual partners should attend for examination and treatment, as otherwise reinfection is very common. All patients with perianal warts should have a proctoscopic examination to exclude rectal involvement. In children with genital warts the possibility of sexual abuse must be considered.

Fig. 6.11 Extensive perivulvar warts. In this situation full gynaecological examination is essential to rule out continuing infection.

HPVs types 16 and 18 are commonly found in genital warts, and there is current controversy about their oncogenic potential.

Pathology

Biopsy is rarely required to confirm the clinical diagnosis. The histopathology is, however, characteristic. Hyperkeratosis and acanthosis are accompanied by large numbers of keratohyalin granules in the Malpighian layer. Some epidermal cells are vacuolated and may also contain basophilic inclusions. The wart virus can be clearly seen and identified by electron microscopy.

Diagnosis

Diagnosis of warts is usually made by the patient. Occasionally, the periungual fibromata of tuberous sclerosis are misdiagnosed as periungual warts, but close examination and a search for other signs of this condition (p. 269) should clarify the situation. Plantar warts may be confused with either corns or, if haemorrhage into the lesion has occurred causing discoloration, with invasive malignant tumours such as malignant melanoma.

Paring down the lesion with a sharp scalpel blade can be of diagnostic help as in plantar warts punctate bleeding points will be seen. In corns one sees only a thickened epidermis while in a malignant tumour, such as melanoma, dark friable vascular tissue will be revealed. If a malignant tumour is suspected the patient should be referred without delay for a diagnostic excision biopsy. It is preferable to excise unnecessarily the occasional plantar wart than to treat a malignant melanoma inappropriately.

Genital warts may be confused with condylomata lata of syphilis and, as both conditions are transmitted by sexual contact, they may coexist. Full serological screening for venereal diseases should therefore be performed routinely on all cases of genital warts.

Treatment

A large proportion of **common warts** will involute spontaneously and therefore either no treatment or placebo treatment for the first 3–4 months after presentation is quite acceptable, particularly in the case of small children. If therapy is considered necessary, a salicylic acid paint (for example 12 per cent salicylic acid, 10 per cent acetone, and collodion to 100 per cent—Salactol, Duofilm) is recommended. Paints containing glutaraldehyde (Glutarol) are also useful. For lesions persisting despite a 3–4 month trial of such paints, cryotherapy with liquid nitrogen, or a slush of carbon dioxide snow and acetone can be used. Warts should be frozen for sufficient time to cause the surrounding skin to develop a white halo. Some discomfort is inevitable, and blistering may develop 24–48 hours after treatment. The procedure should be repeated at 3-weekly intervals until the warts are gone. Curettage, or electrocautery, or diathermy under local anaesthesia are standard methods for dealing with more persistent warts. Radiotherapy has been used in the past, but nowadays is not to be recommended even for persistent lesions.

With all forms of therapy the recurrence rate is relatively high.

Plane warts, particularly on the face, should be treated by bland, non-scarring preparations. Salicylic acid paints may accelerate spontaneous clearance.

For **plantar warts** slightly different methods are more likely to be successful. The first step is to pare away as much of the overlying hard skin as possible, and then apply salicylic acid or gluteraldehyde-containing paint (Salactol, Glutarol), and covering with occlusive plaster. In some countries 25–50 per cent podophyllin in liquid paraffin or white soft paraffin is used. This causes tissue necrosis if an occlusive bandage is kept in place for 10–14 days. The remaining wart virus-infected tissue can be curetted away after this period.

Formalin soaks are also of value. The patient applies a protective layer of Vaseline to the surrounding normal skin, then immerses the wart for 10–20 minutes in a saucer containing 3–6 per cent formalin in an aqueous solution. This is repeated daily, and after 2–3 weeks warts become smaller and desiccated, and can be curetted out with ease and little pain.

Genital warts can be persistent and difficult to treat. Full vaginal and/or rectal examination should be performed to establish the extent of the problem before starting to treat the visible lesions. Cryotherapy can then be commenced, and used weekly or twice weekly for as long as is necessary. This is at present the best method of out-patient management, causing relatively little discomfort. Alternatively, daily applications for 3–4 days of podophyllin 25–50 per cent in soft paraffin is effective, but it leads to considerable maceration and discomfort. It is difficult to use on an out-patient basis.

Situations in which warts must be regarded as a more serious problem are pregnancy and immunosuppression. Young pregnant women with a few mild genital warts tend rapidly to develop large, fungating, cauliflower-like masses of lesions. The use of podophyllin in pregnant women is *not* recommended because of sporadic case reports of fetal damage. Early and efficient treatment of small lesions with cryotherapy is the treatment of choice.

In the immunosuppressed patient warts can grow with alarming speed and give rise to major problems. Children on long-term chemotherapy for leukaemia and other malignancies tend to develop large and very persistent lesions. Such patients should be treated promptly and effectively as spontaneous resolution is most unlikely to occur. It is also good practice to examine such children for warts prior to commencing chemotherapy and treat any lesions before further chemotherapy-induced immunosuppression develops. Transplant recipients tend to be very difficult to treat once they develop warts, and it is good practice to vigorously treat all warts prior to transplantation to prevent future problems. Very persistent warts in transplant patients may require specialist measures such as intralesional bleomycin or systemic interferon.

Treating warts in small children is painful and not always essential as the majority will resolve spontaneously. Allow time for this.

Key Points

Molluscum contagiosum and orf are caused by a pox virus.

Definition

An infectious cutaneous lesion caused by a pox virus.

This benign, but troublesome condition is a common cause for dermatological out-patient referral in the under-fives, and occasionally in older children and adults. Multiple lesions are common in young children, but in adults isolated lesions, sometimes of considerable size, are more common.

Pathology

Biopsy is rarely required and is usually performed on a large isolated lesion to exclude other more serious conditions. The histological changes are confined to the epidermis and consist of acanthosis, hyperkeratosis, and an increase in the numbers of keratohyalin granules. As epidermal cells in the centre of the lesion are destroyed they are replaced by large, amorphous, eosinophilic structures, the molluscum bodies, which are the histological hallmark of this condition.

Clinical features

The lesions are most commonly seen on the face and neck, although the trunk may also be involved. The lesions are elevated, smooth, reddish papules and all have a small central punctum which is an important diagnostic point to be sought (Fig. 6.12 and 6.13). Troublesome lesions may develop around the eyelids and at the vermilion border of the lip. In adults, isolated lesions may develop on any body site and in recent years crops of mollusca on genital skin have been seen more commonly.

Diagnosis and treatment

Diagnosis is usually straightforward, but an isolated lesion may not be recognized until histological examination of curettings or of a biopsy.

Fig. 6.12 Molluscum contagiosum. Note central punctum, seen best on the largest lesion.

Fig. 6.13 Molluscum contagiosum. Note cluster of pearly lesions with central umbilication.

The aim of treatment is to stimulate an inflammatory reaction in the dermis underlying the lesion. This can be achieved by puncturing the lesions individually with a curette or forceps, and applying iodine to the area. Liquid nitrogen or carbon dioxide/acetone slush can also be used, but are less effective.

Orf

Definition
A rapidly growing solitary cutaneous lesion caused by a pox virus.

Clinical features
The infection is contracted through contact with sheep, either directly or indirectly from barbed wire, grass, or other material adjacent to the animals. It is easily and quickly recognized by agricultural workers, country dwellers, and veterinary surgeons, but may dismay and alarm a town dweller who develops a rapidly expanding lesion on his hand 2 weeks after a visit to a farm in the country.

After an incubation period of 7–10 days a red papule develops, commonly on the sides of the fingers, rapidly grows, and finally reaches a size of 5–10 cm, with a central necrotic or bullous area (Fig. 6.14). Lymphangitis, local lymphadenopathy, and fever are not uncommon. Spontaneous recovery takes place and one attack confers subsequent immunity.

Treatment
A broad spectrum systemic antibiotic is commonly given orally for 5–7 days, for example flucloxacillin. Topical antibiotics, such as 3 per cent aureomycin ointment, may also be used.

Fig. 6.14 Orf. Note large pustular lesion which has developed rapidly on the hand of a town dweller who had helped a sheep caught in barbed wire 10 days previously.

Key Points

Primary infection with *Herpes virus hominis* type 1 is almost universal early in life.

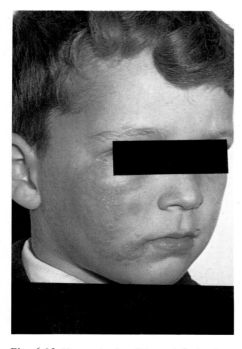

Fig. 6.15 Herpes simplex. Primary infection in an 8-year-old boy.

Herpes simplex

Definition

A cutaneous infection due to *Herpes virus hominis*.

Two types of *H. hominis* virus are currently recognized. Type 1 is the variety mainly responsible for recurrent 'cold sores' in the upper lip area, and type 2 is usually associated with genital herpes lesions. Carcinoma of the cervix is commoner in women with a high titre of antibody to the type 2 virus, but no putative or proven association with malignancy has yet been reported with the type 1 virus.

Primary infection with type 1 virus is almost universal in childhood or early adult life and is usually subclinical. Thereafter, most people have no further problems, but a few have exacerbations of *H. hominis* infection, usually on the upper lip, often in association with other viral infections. No specific immunological difference between these individuals and those without recurrent herpes simplex has yet been identified.

Pathology

The epidermis shows the significant changes. Gross intracellular oedema leads to balloon degeneration of the infected epidermal cells. The nuclei of these cells show specific intranuclear inclusions. Large multinucleate giant cells may also be seen in persistent infections.

Clinical features

The characteristic clinical picture of an active, primary *H. hominis* type 1 infection is a miserable, febrile child with a painful ulcerated mouth, and painful enlarged local lymph nodes (Fig. 6.15). The lesions persist for 3–6 days

Fig. 6.16 Herpetic whitlow. Very often these lesions are regarded as bacterial and lanced. Never forget that viruses as well as bacteria can give rise to painful fingers of this type.

and subside spontaneously. They consist of a group of small blisters on the skin surface as well as on buccal mucous membrane. If the cornea is involved, immediate ophthalmological care should be instituted, as corneal scarring and ulceration are common sequelae. *Herpetic whitlow* or inoculation herpes simplex is common in hospital workers and results from the virus entering through a small abrasion, usually on the fingers (Fig. 6.16). Frequently misdiagnosed as a pyogenic lesion, it consists of a painful, indurated, and tender area, topped by blisters which initially are filled with clear fluid. Occasionally, primary infection on the trunk may have a linear distribution and cause confusion with herpes zoster.

Recurrent herpes simplex attacks begin with a tingling sensation, and then tender, painful lesions appear, usually on the upper lip.

Patients with AIDS may develop very extensive, painful, and persistent H simplex infections usually with herpes simplex type 2.

Diagnosis and treatment

If there is doubt clinically, the most rapid way to confirm the diagnosis is to examine a thick smear from the surface of the lesion in the electron microscope to identify the viral particles. Blood samples can be taken both at the time of presentation and 10–14 days later to demonstrate a rise in titre of antibody to the virus. An alternative rapid diagnostic method for identifying both herpes simplex and herpes zoster is to use a specific fluorescein-labelled antibody directed against the virus in a frozen section from a skin biopsy of the lesion.

Management of severe primary infection is largely supportive, to maintain an adequate fluid balance. If necessary, systemic antibiotics can be administered to control secondary infection.

Recurrent herpes simplex lesions are difficult to prevent. Acyclovir (Zovirax) given orally in doses of 200 mg × 5/day may reduce the severity of recurrent attacks, but only if introduced in the very early stages of the recurrence. In the

Key Points

Topical steroid should not be applied to lesions with actively growing virus.

case of patients who have already had multiple recurrences, 200 mg acyclovir given orally × 2–3/day for several months may reduce the number of recurrences. Topical acyclovir preparations have, in general, been relatively ineffective.

For topical use, 10 per cent povidone iodine paint (Betadine paint, UK) will dry the lesions and reduce secondary bacterial infection. Topical acyclovir is of doubtful value once the infection is well established. Patients with herpes simplex should be warned specifically not to use a topical steroid on the lesions and told to avoid contact with individuals who have atopic eczema.

Herpes simplex infection in the immunosuppressed and in patients with atopic dermatitis can be serious and potentially life-threatening. Hospitalization, supportive care, and full doses of acyclovir, given orally or intravenously, are matters of urgency. It is important to protect these two groups of patients from herpes simplex infection and mothers of children with atopic dermatitis should be warned that persons with cold sores are hazardous to their child.

Herpes zoster (shingles)

Definition

A cutaneous infection caused by the chickenpox virus, *Herpesvirus varicellae.*

Herpes zoster is a disease of adult life and old age, being very rare in children and healthy young adults. As with other viral infections, however, it can develop in a virulent and fulminating form in those who are immunosuppressed either by disease or by therapy. Patients with Hodgkin's disease are particularly prone to develop herpes zoster.

Pathology

As in herpes simplex, the striking histological feature of herpes zoster is balloon degeneration—the presence of grossly swollen, distorted cells in the epidermis. Direct immunofluorescence using antibodies specific for herpes simplex or herpes zoster will differentiate between the two while the infection is at a very early stage. Serology will differentiate from about 14 days after infection.

Clinical features

After prodromal pain, usually in a dermatome distribution, malaise, and sometimes fever, a linear erythematous band develops on this dermatome (Fig. 6.17 and 6.18). Groups of small blisters then develop on the erythema. Some of these may become secondarily infected, and local lymphadenopathy is common. Pain may appear to be out of proportion to the other clinical signs, and when it persists and evolves into post-herpetic neuralgia, it is extremely difficult to treat.

Certain clinical varieties require special management. These include involvement of the ophthalmic division of the trigeminal nerve, leading to ocular damage and the Ramsey–Hunt syndrome when the geniculate ganglia are affected, causing pain and blistering of the external ear. Involvement of the

Fig. 6.17 Herpes zoster. Severe herpes zoster infection involving the trigeminal nerve.

Fig. 6.18 Herpes zoster showing extensive scarring on the shoulder in the dermatomal distribution. This particular individual had extensive post herpetic pain.

first and second sacral ganglia may cause severe ulceration in the genital region and urinary retention. In the elderly, unfit, or immunosuppressed more than one dermatome may be involved.

Diagnosis and treatment

The clinical appearance is usually diagnostic, but occasionally examination of a thick smear in the electron microscope, or immunofluorescence, is required. Treatment of mild cases is symptomatic, and consists of simple analgesics, maintenance of fluid balance, and soothing topical (drying) applications of lotions such as povidone iodine or ichthyol 1 per cent in oily calamine lotion. Topical steroids should *not* be applied to this or to any other lesion in which actively growing virus is present. The lesions will clear in 7–10 days.

In patients with painful and more widespread infection or immuno-suppressed a full course of acyclovir 800 mg × 5/day for 7 days is recommended. There is some evidence that acyclovir will reduce the incidence and severity of post herpetic neuralgia.

The management of post-herpetic neuralgia is unsatisfactory. A 7–10-day course of systemic corticosteroids may help some otherwise healthy patients, but in others the pain is persistent and severe, and neurosurgical intervention may have to be considered.

Spirochaetal Infections

Lyme Disease

Definition

A multisystem disease caused by the spirochaete borrelia and transmitted to man by the tick *Ixodes ricinus*.

Fig. 6.19 Erythema chronicum migrans. Lower leg of a keen hill walker who had been walking in the New Forest one week before the development of this lesion.

Key Points

Fungal infections are caused by yeasts and dermatophytes.

Incidence and aetiology

In the early 1980s a new disease entity and its cause were recognized in the small town of Lyme, Connecticut, USA. Lyme disease develops after a bite from the tick *Ixodes ricinus* which carries the causative organism, the spirochaete, *Borrelia burgdorferi*. These ticks are found in large numbers in the New England woods, in Scandinavia, in Austria, and in wooded parts of the UK. The exact incidence of Lyme disease is not known, but small scale population studies in countries such as Austria suggest, from serological analysis, that up to 25 per cent of the population in these areas have had past exposure and developed an antibody response.

Clinical features

After a tick bite, which the patient may not remember, there is frequently a febrile episode and the patient then develops a red, raised, slowly changing plaque or erythema around the tick bite (Fig. 6.19). This is *erythema chronicum migrans*, the best established dermatological association of Lyme disease. A biopsy of this site and very careful search may reveal the spirochaete in the lesion. Patients will also have circulating antibodies to *Borrelia burgdorferi* but the presence of these antibodies cannot be taken as proof of cause of the cutaneous lesion because of the possibility of previous exposure. A later cutaneous association with Lyme disease is acrodermatitis chronica atrophicans.

Non-dermatological manifestations of Lyme disease include musculoskeletal and neurological problems, including meningitis and isolated nerve palsies.

Treatment

Therapy for erythema chronicum migrans and any other dermatological problem thought to be associated with Lyme disease is either oral penicillin or tetracycline in full doses for a minimum of 2 weeks. Repeated courses may be required.

Fungal Infections

Two main groups of fungi infect man. These are the *Candida* group of yeasts and the *dermatophytes*. *Candida albicans* is the most common species responsible for human infection and of the dermatophytes, *Trichophyton rubrum, Trichophyton mentagrophytes* var. *interdigitale, Trichophyton tonsurans*, and *Epidermophyton floccosum* are the commonest pathogens in the UK. All these dermatophytes are transmitted directly from one human host to another. However, humans can contract animal ringworm from domestic animals, the usual dermatophytes responsible being *Microsporum canis* and *Trichophyton verrucosum*.

Pityriasis versicolor, due to a yeast, *Malassezia furfur*, is a superficial infection and will be discussed in this section.

Candida infections (candidosis, thrush)

Candida albicans is a normal commensal of the gastro-intestinal tract, and can be grown from apparently healthy, normal mouths and perianal skin. In the very young, the elderly, and in those whose natural microbiological flora has been disturbed by disease, or by therapy such as antibiotics, it may become a pathogen. It can be a serious and resistant problem in those with HIV.

Pathology

Candida albicans exists both as yeasts and in hyphal form. In pathological conditions budding yeasts and pseudohyphae are easily seen, and best visualized by staining with periodic acid Schiff (PAS). They lie in the stratum corneum. Persistent lesions may be associated with abscess formation, acanthosis, and, in more severe cases, with a granulomatous reaction.

Clinical features

Cutaneous lesions due to *Candida albicans* present in infants as napkin candidosis and in the elderly as intertrigo affecting the submammary folds, the axillae, and the groins (Fig. 6.20). In both situations the lesions are a glazed brick-red and are characterized by 'satellite lesions' and occasionally pustules around the main area of involvement. These are isolated individual lesions which have the same colour and appearance as the main lesion. Painful fissures frequently develop in the affected body folds and may be resistant to therapy.

In people with occupations which involve wet work, candidal paronychia is an occupational hazard. Initially, the protective cuticle between nail and nail fold is lost, allowing Candida to invade the space thus created. The resulting inflammation produces a 'bolstered' posterior nail fold from which beads of pus can be expressed.

Chronic candidal granuloma, most commonly on the lips, may develop in patients who have a long history of candidosis. This consists of a firm, indurated area and must not be mistaken for a developing malignancy.

Lesions due to *Candida* on the mucous membranes may involve the mouth, the urogenital area, the oesophagus, and the alimentary tract. Oral candidosis

Fig. 6.20 Inframammary candidosis in an obese diabetic patient.

produces adherent white patches on the tongue and inner surfaces of the cheeks. If scraped off, a raw bleeding area will be revealed. In the elderly these lesions are fairly common under dental plates and may be very difficult to cure as the plate itself is frequently colonized by the organism. Candidal vulvovaginitis causes an irritable erythema associated with a copious discharge. There is no evidence that oral contraceptives predispose to this condition, but pregnant and diabetic women are more at risk. *Candida* infecting the bronchial or alimentary mucous membranes is less common but should always be borne in mind when infants with napkin *Candida* have persistent diarrhoea.

Generalized systemic infections due to *Candida* are rare and usually associated with immunosuppression or antibiotic therapy. Chronic mucocutaneous candidosis is rare, but of great interest to dermatologists and immunologists as it is a model for establishing the relative value of cell-mediated and humoral immunity in the host response to *Candida*.

Diagnosis and treatment

All lesions thought to be due to *Candida* should be swabbed and examined for the presence of the organism. In typical cases this serves merely to confirm a clinical impression, but in less classic presentations it is essential. It must be remembered, however, that the presence of the organism does not automatically imply a pathogenetic role, and also that *Candida* may colonize a pre-existing skin condition such as seborrhoeic dermatitis and cause an opportunistic secondary infection rather than primary disease.

Treatment depends firstly on altering the damp, moist, warm microclimate in which *Candida* thrives. Thus, napkin candidosis will not clear as long as the infant is wrapped in damp napkins. Similarly, obese females with pendulous breasts will retain their inframammary *Candida* as long as the two apposing skin surfaces remain in close contact. Soaks or swabs should therefore be used to separate skin folds in such situations.

For patients with an intact immune system, the choice of therapy lies between nystatin-containing preparations and imidazoles. Nystatin is available as an oral suspension, and in pessary, cream, gel, and ointment formulation. It has a well-established safety record and is the preparation of choice for use in infants. Imidazoles include clotrimazole (Canesten, UK; Lotrimin, USA) cream, econazole (Spectazole, US), miconazole (Daktarin) sulconazole and ketoconazole. Ketoconazole appears to have greater activity against *Candida* than the other imidazoles.

Candida paronychia is relatively slow to respond to therapy, but good results will be achieved by instructing the patient to work nystatin ointment well into the nail fold and to keep the hands dry. If working conditions necessitate rubber gloves, a separate pair of cotton gloves should be worn next to the skin and changed frequently. 'Denture mouth' due to *Candida* requires concomitant treatment of the mouth with nystatin suspension, miconazole gel, or amphotericin B lozenges and also nightly soaking of the dentures in an antifungal solution.

Infants with persistent napkin *Candida* should be given oral nystatin drops as a high proportion will have involvement of the alimentary tract.

Topical steroids are an excellent growth medium for *Candida* and are contraindicated.

Persistent and severe candidal infection is a particular problem in patients who are therapeutically immunosuppressed or in those whose immune system is severely depressed as in HIV infection. In those situations the use of oral imidazoles such as fluconazole (Diflucan, UK) or itraconazole (Sporanox UK) as a prophylactic measure appears effective and safe. Very short courses of these oral imidazoles are also extremely effective in eradicating persistent genital candidosis in otherwise healthy non-immunosuppressed individuals.

Persistent candidal infection is a sign of immunosuppression, not a disease *per se*. Investigate your patient for underlying problems.

Dermatophyte infections

Definition

Cutaneous lesions due to dermatophytes, presenting most commonly as athlete's foot, nail infections, tinea corporis, and scalp ringworm.

Pathology

These pathogenic fungi inhabit the keratinized tissue of skin, hair, and nails, and generally do not invade living tissue. In active infections they are seen as branched hyphae. They grow down the pilosebaceous follicles towards the hair bulb, but are arrested before reaching the bulb itself and fan out to form multiple hyphal fronds known as **Adamson's fringe**. The hair shaft is invaded.

Dermatophytes can be seen on **direct examination** by taking skin scrapings (p. 34) or nail clippings from the affected area and mounting them on a slide with coverslip in 10–20 per cent potassium hydroxide, which is gently warmed and examined microscopically. To identify the particular dermatophyte present it is necessary to culture the samples for up to 3 weeks on a suitable medium such as Sabouraud's. These techniques, rather than biopsy, constitute the correct method of identifying fungi, but if it is necessary to look for fungi in a histological section it should be stained with periodic acid Schiff (PAS) or methenamine silver to show them in the stratum corneum.

Clinical features

Tinea pedis (athlete's foot)

This common condition is found in adolescents and young adults, particularly those who use communal changing facilities, showers, and swimming pools. The usual site of infection is the toe webs, especially the fourth, where moist, white 'blotting-paper' skin will be seen. Pruritus is common. The instep (Fig. 6.21), and in persistent cases the nails, may also be involved and therapy then poses considerable difficulties.

Fig. 6.21 Tinea pedis involving the instep and heel. *Trichophyton rubrum* was cultured from scrapings.

The organisms most commonly found are *Trichophyton rubrum, Trichophyton mentagrophytes* var. *interdigitale*, and *Epidermophyton floccosum*.

Tinea corporis (ringworm)

Infection of the trunk frequently begins in the body folds such as the groins or axillae and presents as an itchy, erythematous area with a raised advancing edge. Scrapings will be most likely to yield positive results if taken from this edge.

Diagnosis is not always straightforward. Isolated scaling lesions on the trunk may resemble psoriasis (Figs 6.22 and 6.23). If tinea corporis has been treated with topical steroids, its presentation may be atypical. Persistent hand dermati-

Figs 6.22 and 6.23 Scaling lesions on the trunk. Mycological examination showed both to be due to fungal infection. Note the superficial similarity to areas of psoriasis.

tis may be due to dermatophytes, most commonly *Trichophyton rubrum*, in which case the palm is dry with itchy, scaly creases. Mycological examination should be routine in such circumstances.

Dermatophyte infection of the hair shaft on the scalp or beard area may be due to *T. tonsurans, M. canis, T. rubrum*, or *T. verrucosum* (Fig. 6.24). Usually, the first sign is a well-circumscribed pruritic scaling area of hair loss, with a variable inflammatory response. Suspected hair infection should always be examined under Wood's light (ultraviolet light > 365 nm) as lesions due to *M. canis* and *M. audouinii* will show a diagnostic brilliant green fluorescence. Those due to *Trichophyton* species do not give rise to this degree of fluorescence, although *T. schoenleinii* causes a dull green fluorescence and gives rise to the distinctive clinical entity called **favus**. Favus is now most common in North America, around the Mediterranean, and in the Middle East. The characteristic features are extensive— even complete—hair loss, scalp atrophy leading to permanent alopecia, and the presence of adherent scales (scutulae) on the remaining hairs.

Infection of the hair shaft with *T. verrucosum* may cause a very brisk inflammatory reaction, termed a **kerion** (Fig. 6.25), seen commonly in children after contact with cattle or other domestic animals. There is a dramatic, acute folliculitis with pustules and swelling forming a boggy mass on the scalp. Hair loss and eventual scarring alopecia are common, but one attack usually confers subsequent immunity.

In persistent foot dermatitis *always* exclude a fungal cause by sending scrapings for mycology.

Fig.6.24 Tinea capitis. Brilliant green fluorescence was seen under Wood's light and *Microsporum audouinii* isolated in culture.

Diagnosis and treatment

Direct microscopy of scrapings in potassium hydroxide and the use of Wood's light in the clinic or consulting room will immediately confirm the clinical diagnosis in a high proportion of dermatophyte infections. The remainder will require culture of skin scrapings or nail clippings. Any persistent scaling lesions should be scraped and examined in this way as atypical fungal infections may mimic psoriasis, seborrhoeic dermatitis, or mycosis fungoides. Over-diagnosis of dermatophyte infections may also occur, particularly in the case of lesions of the feet when the true cause may be simple maceration from hyperhidrosis or allergic contact dermatitis to footwear. Any persistent lesions on the feet which do not respond to antifungal therapy should be carefully reviewed, particularly if there is no involvement of the interdigital clefts.

Cutaneous dermatophyte infections can be treated with topical or oral preparations. Topical preparations include the allylamines (terbinafine, Lamisil) and the imidazoles, which are available as creams, including sulconazole (Exelderm), UK; miconazole (Daktarin), UK; Monistat derm USA; and ketoconazole (Nizoral), UK and USA.

Oral griseofulvin, and oral terbinafine (Lamisil) which are effective against dermatophytes, but not *Candida* species, should be reserved for more severe cutaneous infections involving body sites other than, or in addition to, the interdigital clefts. They are, however, the treatment of choice for widespread or

Fig. 6.25 Extensive kerion in an immigrant child.

persistent tinea corporis, tinea capitis, and tinea unguium. The dose is 1 g of griseofulvin daily for adults. This should be give orally during a fatty meal. Duration of treatment varies with site of involvement, but in general 4–6 weeks for scalp and body lesions.

Terbinafine is fungicidal and is effective in treating both finger and toenails which were previously resistant to therapy. It should be given in a dose of 250 mg/day for 6 weeks and the course may be repeated once. Thereafter topical terbinafine can applied to the nail bed area as the new nail grows in.

Prevention of tinea pedis can to a large extent be achieved by simple hygiene, footbaths, and the use of an antifungal dusting powder after using communal baths and showers.

Pityriasis versicolor

Definition

A persistent, usually asymptomatic, fungal infection of the trunk due to *Malassezia furfur*.

This infection is relatively common in tropical countries and is seen with increased frequency in Britain during spells of hot humid weather. The causative organism is known as *Pityrosporum orbiculare* in its yeast-like form, and as *Malassezia furfur* when it becomes hyphal. These hyphae and yeasts can be recognized in skin scrapings, or Scotch tape strippings, or on biopsy material using PAS stain. The hyphae are found in the horny layers and there is little underlying reaction.

Clinical features

The lesions are asymptomatic, mainly on the trunk and proximal parts of the limbs, with a fine superficial scale seen best after gently scraping the surface with a fingernail. Untanned, white, Caucasian skin shows an increase in pigmentation in the affected areas with a yellowish-brown scale, but in darker skin or heavily tanned skin there is depigmentation. The overall effect is a dappled appearance (Fig. 6.26, 6.27, and 6.28).

Diagnosis and treatment

Skin scrapings for direct microscopy and examination under Wood's light for pale yellow fluorescence can both be used to identify the organism. Vitiligo (p. 199) is frequently confused with pityriasis versicolor and scrapings should be taken from all atypical cases.

Many topical preparations have been recommended for therapy, but recurrences are common. The current treatment of choice is a topical imidazole. Clotrimazole solution, miconazole cream, and econazole cream and lotion are all effective.

Figs 6.26, 6.27 and 6.28 Lesions of pityriasis versicolor showing increase in pigmentation in white skinned individuals but conversely a decrease in darker skinned individuals.

Fig. 6.29 Cutaneous leishmaniasis on the wrist in an individual normally resident in the UK 8 weeks after visiting the Middle East.

Protozoal Infection

Leishmaniasis

Definition

Cutaneous or systemic infection caused by the parasite leishmania, and transmitted by a bite from a sand fly.

The pathology of the type of leishmania infection most commonly seen in the UK is a superficial granuloma. Careful search will reveal leishman Donovan bodies in the cells of the granuloma.

Clinical features

Leishmaniasis is a major problem in South America, Africa, and southern Mediterranean countries. The reader is advised to consult a tropical dermatology text for a detailed account. The most likely presentation in the UK is a crusted sore on the face, hand, or leg 6–8 weeks after returning from an endemic area (Fig. 6.29). Cases have recently been reported in holiday-makers after returning from Spain. The patient may not remember the sand fly bite.

Diagnosis

Diagnosis is based on the history, histology, and, if required a positive leishmanin test, an intradermal injection of heat-killed organisms.

Treatment

In healthy individuals, cutaneous leishmaniasis frequently resolves spontaneously. Cryotherapy is also effective and, for persistent cases, oral pentavalent antimony (Pentostam) is required.

Cutaneous Infestations

The commonest infestations in man are due to lice and scabies.

Scabies

Definition

A persistent pruritic skin eruption caused by cutaneous infestation with the mite *Sarcoptes scabei*.

The female (Fig. 6.30) inhabits a burrow in the stratum corneum and eventually dies after laying her eggs there. The eggs hatch and the new generation matures in 14 days, when the cycle is repeated.

The incidence of scabies varies on a world scale with hygiene, housing conditions, and population movements. Epidemics have been associated with

Key Points

Remember that scabies infection in those who have a high standard of hygiene can be very subtle.

Fig. 6.30 The female scabies mite or *Acarus*.

world wars, and recent local increases in incidence in Europe have been attributed to changing social habits and increasing body contact. Frequently, whole households are infested, although only one member may complain of symptoms.

Pathology

A local hypersensitivity reaction to the female scabies mite is assumed to cause release of inflammatory mediators, giving rise to severe and persistent itch.

If scabies lesions are biopsied, usually in error, the female mite and her eggs may be seen in a burrow high in the stratum corneum. Occasionally, nodular lesions persist long after successful therapy and these consist of a chronic inflammatory reaction with many lymphocytes in the dermis.

Clinical features

Patients complain bitterly of severe and persistent itch, worse after bathing and at night. In those who have a high standard of personal hygiene, lesions may be very sparse, but the classical sites of involvement are the finger webs, the sides of the fingers (Fig. 6.31), the flexor aspects of the wrists, the points of the elbows, the anterior axillary fold, the periumbilical area, the penile or scrotal skin in males (Figs 6.32 and 6.33), and the areolae of the nipple in females. In infants who are not yet walking, striking involvement of the soles is common (Fig. 6.34). The individual lesions may seem superficially to be excoriated papules, but on closer inspection a linear burrow may be seen extending from this papule. The mite can frequently be extracted from this burrow with a needle, and painting the area with indian ink, then washing off the excess on the skin surface will demonstrate dramatically the extent of the burrows. In long-standing cases secondary infection with pustule formation, crusting is common, and nodular lesions which persist for months after successful therapy may be seen. These are commonest on the buttocks and the male genitalia.

Fig. 6.31 Scabetic lesions on the hands. An acarus was extracted from the raised lesion on the third (middle) finger.

Figs 6.32 and 6.33 Scabies involving the wrists and genital area respectively.

A moist oozing infected dermatitis may develop on top of scabetic burrows and dermatitic lesions on scabetic sites of predilection should be very carefully examined for underlying burrows.

Diagnosis and treatment

In all cases demonstration of the acarus by extracting it from a burrow should be attempted as this is the cardinal diagnostic test. The most common mistake is to misdiagnose scabies either as contact dermatitis or as dermatitis herpetiformis. All cases of presumed scabies in which the acarus has not been identified, and which do not respond to therapy, should be reassessed and biopsy considered.

The most useful acaricides are 1 per cent gamma benzene hexachloride (lindane—Quellada), malathion (Derbac M, Suleo M), and permethrin (Lyclear).

Fig. 6.34 Scabetic lesions in an infant aged 9 months. Note the striking involvement of the soles of the feet.

Sulphur preparations, such as 2.5 per cent sulphur ointment or monosulfiram (Tetmosol), are recommended in many centres for infants because of the risk of percutaneous absorption of the first two preparations. It is essential that the entire body from the neck to the soles of the feet be treated and that the hands are re-treated during the course of the 24 hours for which the preparation should remain on the skin. A 2-inch paintbrush or cotton wool swabs are useful applicators. After 24 hours the application can be washed off in a hot bath. If it is considered necessary, this procedure can be repeated once or twice but if instructions are properly followed, this should not be necessary. Twenty-four hours after the last application the patient should bathe, and all clothing and bed linen be washed. Boiling or fumigation is not required. Pruritus may continue for a few days even after successful therapy, and crotamiton cream (Eurax, UK) will minimize this.

All household and other close contacts of a confirmed case of scabies should be warned that they are likely to be infested, and should be treated at the same time as the patient, even if they are asymptomatic. The usual cause of persistent scabies is either inadequate application of topical therapy or reinfestation from contacts. Written instructions to patients on how to treat themselves and their families will increase the likelihood of the correct procedures being followed.

Pediculosis capitis

Pediculosis capitis is a relatively common problem in schoolchildren in various parts of the world, and at present it is prevalent in certain large cities in the UK. Pediculosis corporis is less common, and is most frequently seen in vagrants and others living in very poor social circumstances.

The well-known nit is a head-louse egg, stuck firmly to scalp hair by its capsule. Nits may look like fine adherent dandruff particles. There are no associated symptoms until the louse hatches, when an irritant dermatitis on the scalp develops. Scratching leads to secondary impetiginization, particularly at the nape of the neck and behind the ears.

Diagnosis and treatment

Identification of the nit or of the adult head louse with the naked eye is straightforward. Shaving the head is not required, but cutting the hair short will facilitate treatment and lessen the risk of reinfestation. Brushing of the hair with a fine brush will result in nits sticking to the brush (Fig. 6.35).

Malathion (Derbac M, Suleo M) and permethrin (Lyclear) are all useful preparations at present, but resistance is developing, and if a patient does not respond to one of these, an alternative should be substituted. These should be applied to the entire scalp and left for 12–24 hours, the hair should then be shampooed and dead nits combed out. Treatment may have to be repeated after 7–10 days in a few cases. As with scabies, all affected family members should be examined and treated simultaneously if required. Other contacts in schools should also be checked for infestation, but a current common source of reinfection in children in the UK is from older household contacts such as grandparents.

Fig. 6.35 Brushings showing nits firmly adherent to the bristles of the brush.

Pediculosis corporis (body lice)

Patients infested with body lice usually present with pruritus, excoriations, and secondary infection. Weals and erythematous macules may also be seen, but the source of the problem should be sought and identified by examining the seams of clothing worn next to the skin. This is the site where they are likely to be found. In chronic cases striking pigmentation may be observed on the trunk and limbs.

Treatment

Infested clothing should be removed and fumigated with malathion or an alternative parasiticide. The patient should be examined for concomitant infestation with scabies and head lice. One treatment with 0.5 per cent malathion to the body is recommended, followed by the use of a topical steroid/antibiotic preparation to accelerate relief of symptoms.

Pediculosis pubis

The pubic louse is transmitted by close body contact and qualifies as a sexually transmitted disease. Patients complain of pruritus and have the characteristic blue-black 'dots' in their pubic hair. These are the pubic lice, engorged after sucking blood from their host.

Treatment

One or two applications of gamma benzene hexachloride lotion will kill the lice. Sexual partners should be treated simultaneously.

The Sexually Transmitted Diseases

In most European countries, dermatology and venereology are combined specialties, but in the UK the two subjects are divided into separate specialties. In practice, however, patients with venereal disease may well present initially to a dermatological clinic. A brief mention of the cutaneous manifestations of syphilis and gonorrhoea is therefore included in this chapter. For a more comprehensive account the reader is referred to a specialist textbook.

Syphilis

The patient with syphilis may present with dermatological manifestations in any of the three stages of infection. In the primary stage there is a **primary chancre** at the site of sexual contact and from it the causative organism, *Treponema pallidum*, can be isolated. Local lymphadenopathy is common. Four to eight weeks after an untreated primary chancre, secondary syphilis will develop. The dermatological reaction consists of a maculopapular, sometimes lichenoid, rash which affects the whole body including the palms, soles, and mucous membranes. It is generally asymptomatic. Tertiary syphilis is fortunately much rarer than the other stages, but may present to the dermatologist as an isolated, painless, ulcerating lesion, a **gumma**.

The primary chancre

One to four weeks after infection a moist, ulcerating lesion develops on or near genital mucosa. The ulcer has a sharply demarcated edge, and is both indurated and infiltrated. As serology does not become positive until about 4 weeks after contact, all serological studies at this stage may be negative, but *T. pallidum* can be identified by dark-field illumination of a thick smear from the ulcer. Untreated, 20–30 per cent of these patients will develop secondary syphilis.

Secondary syphilis

As secondary syphilis develops 4–8 weeks after primary infection, the primary chancre may still be visible when secondary lesions appear (Fig. 6.36). These are small maculopapules seen on the trunk and limbs, associated with generalized lymphadenopathy, and, if profuse, with **condylomata lata** on the genital mucosa. Lesions on the palms (Fig. 6.37) and soles are important in aiding clinical distinction from other dermatological disorders, such as pityriasis rosea and seborrhoeic dermatitis. Loss of scalp hair and eyebrows may be present, and the pattern of loss is described as 'moth-eaten'.

During this period all patients will have positive serology. *T. pallidum* may be identified in lesions, particularly of the mucosa, and a biopsy will show a perivascular infiltrate, often with many plasma cells, and endarteritis of the small vessels. In cases with untreated lesions, oedema is a common feature. The histological changes are non-specific, although suggestive, and therefore serology must be used for confirmation.

Key Points

Do not forget that syphilis can still be the great imitator.

Fig. 6.36 Macular eruption of secondary syphilis. Lesions may also be seen on the palms of the hands.

Fig. 6.37 Secondary syphilis showing typical eruption on the palms of the hands.

Tertiary syphilis

Cutaneous lesions of tertiary syphilis can appear after a latent period of many years, or even decades. At this stage serology is not reliable. Histologically, there is expansion of granulation tissue, stimulated by the presence of *T. pallidum*, through the dermis and epidermis, leading to ulceration. This is seen clinically as a **gumma**, a painless lesion whose healing is slow and incomplete, with scarring. On the oral mucosa this will ulcerate the soft palate, leading to perforation.

Treatment

Patients with primary or secondary syphilis should be treated with large doses of penicillin G. Commonly, 3–5 megaunits over 3–4 days are used. Sexual contacts should be traced and treated simultaneously.

Gonorrhoea

Cutaneous manifestations of infection with *Neisseria gonorrhoeae* are most commonly superficial erosions on the genital mucous membrane. They appear up to 14 days after sexual contact, and are associated with urethritis and a urethral discharge in men. Women, however, may be asymptomatic. The organisms can be identified on thick smears from the affected area.

Treatment

High doses of penicillin and contact tracing are the important points in management.

Reiter's syndrome

The triad of arthritis, urethritis, and conjunctivitis is known as Reiter's syndrome. A proportion of patients have, in addition, gastrointestinal symptoms. Cutaneous involvement can occur and consists of heaped-up scaling lesions on the feet (termed **keratoderma blenorrhagica**) circinate balanitis, and occasionally lesions on the oral mucous membrane. No causative organism has yet been identified, and there is debate as to whether it should be grouped with sexually transmitted disease or with psoriasis as the lesions on the feet are strikingly similar to psoriasis both clinically and histologically (p. 48).

Treatment

Cutaneous lesions respond to conventional topical psoriasis therapy (p. 54) and the urogenital lesions to systemic tetracycline.

Dermatological complications of infection with the human immunodeficiency virus (HIV 1)

Infection with HIV 1 can be divided into three distinct phases:

(1) **subclinical asymptomatic infection;**

(2) **ARC** or **Aids Related Complex** of weight loss, lymphadenopathy, and frequently one or more of the cutaneous problems listed in Table 6.1;

(3) **Full-blown AIDS** or acquired immunodeficiency syndrome.

Several of the conditions listed in Table 6.1 may coexist in these patients. The majority of the cutaneous complications of HIV 1 infection and their persistence are related to the loss of cell-mediated immunity associated with the condition. This is due to the affinity of the virus for the CD4$^+$ helper T-cell subpopulation and the subsequent gross depletion of these lymphocytes.

It is important to note that, with the exception of **hairy oral leucoplakia**, none of the dermatological problems associated with HIV 1 infection are specific. However, persistent oral candidosis or severe and recurrent genital herpes simplex infection may be the first clinical sign of HIV infection. The possibility that patients with such problems may be in one of the high-risk groups should

Key Points

> Persistent oral candidosis or recurrent genital herpes simplex infection may be the first sign of HIV infection.

Figs 6.38 and 6.39 Patient who is HIV positive with Kaposi's sarcoma. Distant and close-up views showing bluish red nodules. Reproduced by kind permission of Dr Dermot Kennedy.

Table 6.1.
Dermatological complications of HIV 1 infection

Hairy oral leucoplakia

Persistent viral warts and molluscum contagiosum

Persistent or recurrent herpes simplex section

Severe and recurrent candidosis

Seborrhoeic dermatitis-like lesions

Acute onset psoriasis

Severe adverse drug reactions, notably to Septrin

Kaposi's sarcoma

be considered. If indicated, counselling and testing for the HIV viruses should be offered.

Patients with known established HIV infection frequently develop associated dermatological problems. Oral acyclovir may be required prophylactically to prevent recurrences of herpes simplex and oral imidazoles such as fluconazole or itraconazole may be needed to control or prevent candidosis.

Kaposi's sarcoma was noted in some of the earliest patients with AIDS. This is a multifocal malignancy of the capillary endothelium and is recognized clinically as multiple bruise-like areas on any body site, commonly the face and the oral cavity, including the hard palate (Figs 6.38 and 6.39). Temporary control of the lesions can often be achieved with either chemotherapy or localized radiotherapy but the condition tends to recur.

Discussion of problem cases

Case 6.1

In the child with atopic dermatitis, deterioration in his condition could be due to exacerbation of dermatitis, to secondary infection with herpes simplex causing eczema herpeticum, or to secondary infection with staphylococcal impetigo. Exacerbation of atopic dermatitis would be associated, usually, with pruritus and a generalized flare. The child is not seen to be unduly itchy and the lesions on his knees are unchanged. Eczema herpeticum must be excluded in this situation, but is unlikely because the child is not generally unwell. Viral swabs should, however, be taken.

Both the history and the clinical description strongly suggest secondary staphyloccal impetigo. Bacterological swabs confirmed this diagnosis, as a very heavy growth of staph aureus was obtained on culture. Remember that a light growth of staph. can be difficult to interpret as most children with atopic dermatitis have some colonization with staph aureus, but this does not necessarily cause clinical deterioration.

The child was given systemic flucloxacillin syrup for 5 days and topical mupirocin(Bactroban) ointment. After this time, the skin on his face showed marked improvement.

Case 6.2

Psoriasis rarely occurs as an isolated patch, particularly on an atypical site such as the thigh. The most common condition confused with psoriasis as an isolated patch is Bowen's disease or intraepidermal carcinoma in situ (page 289). However, the site and duration of the plaque make Bowen's disease unlikely. A biopsy showed non-caseating granulomas and this, together with the history and clinical appearance, suggested the diagnosis of lupus vulgarus.

Full antituberculous therapy was commenced and over a 9 month period the lesion slowly improved with, of course, no change in the central scarring.

It is possible that this patient had contact with bovine tuberculosis during her childhood on a farm and this gave rise to her problem. Further questioning about her family history also yielded the information that a younger sister had been treated in the past for pulmonary tuberculosis.

Case 6.3

Loss of normal pigmentation is most commonly due to vitiligo (page 199). However, loss of pigment can cause considerable concern to those from India and Asia because of the possibility of leprosy as the depigmentation associated with tublerculoid leprosy is well recognized in these countries. This child showed no evidence of nerve hypertrophy, and no loss of sensation in the depigmented area, both of which would have suggested a diagnosis of leprosy. After a discussion with the parents, a small punch biopsy was taken from the depigmented area and showed only loss of melanocytes with no evidence of granulomas in the underlying dermis. This confirmed the clinical diagnosis of vitiligo, and a moderate potency steroid was prescribed. Over a 6 month period there was no further loss of pigment at the edge of the lesion, and the parents felt there had been a slight improvement in the depigmented area with slight recovery of normal pigmentation in that site.

Case 6.4

In this situation, vigorous treatment of warts in all body sites before transplant and the necessary immunosupression which it entails is very strongly recommended. If patients have warts at the time of receiving their transplant, the warts tend to grow exuberantly when immunosuppressive therapy of any type is introduced. Thereafter they can be very difficult if not impossible to eradicate.

An additional reason for treating warts prior to transplantation is the possible potential for malignant change. Transplant recipients are well recognized as having a higher incidence of non-melanoma skin cancers, mainly squamous cell carcinoma, than the general population, and there is some concern that the types of human papilloma virus found in the transplant population have a higher proportion of the oncogenic types of HPV than in the normal population.

This girl had vigorous treatment with liquid nitrogen fortnightly for 6 weeks to both hand and genital warts and was free of warts when a kidney became available for her 11 weeks later.

Case 6.5

Allergy to footware is not uncommon, but would be unlikely to be unilateral or to involve the calf rather than the dorsum of the foot. The more likely explanation is a bite causing secondary infection. However, the extent of the erythema and the fact that the patient was a reasonably accurate historian tells you that the area of erythema is moving day by day suggests the diagnosis of erythema chronicum migrans. This is the main cutaneous feature of Lyme disease or infection with *Borrelia burgdorferi*, a result of a tick bite. A biopsy was compatible with this diagnosis although a very careful search down a microscope showed no evidence of *Borrelia*. The patient was given a 2 week course of oral tetracycline and a moderate potency steroid antibiotic combination (Trimovate). His lesion cleared within 4 weeks.

Would serology be of value here? If the diagnosis of Lyme disease had not been made, and treatment instituted, what other organs would be at risk?

Case 6.6

The history strongly suggests an infective cause. If a detergent were responsible, the entire population of the home would be likely to be affected. Instead it is a small group of people in a close environment within the home who appear to have the problem.

Possibilities here would include a fungal infection and also scabies. Scrapings were taken from the skin of all patients complaining of itch. No fungi were seen on direct microscopy, but the scabies mite was identified in very large numbers. This suggested that the problem was an outbreak of so-called Norwegian or epidemic scabies. The lack of classic burrows on the skin of these patients may be partly due to thin skin in the elderly, and partly due to the fact that the mite is proliferating on the skin surface.

All residents of the home and all staff were treated with Lindane (Quellada), and all clothing and laundry washed appropriately—a major task.

What would you plan to do about the nurse who has gone on holiday? How would you approach the problem of contact tracing relatives who visit the home?

Projects

1. Run a literature search on Lyme Disease reviews and study them. The early papers show very well how even in the 1980s it has been possible to identify a new disease as a result of careful clinical observation and elegant epidemiological detective work. Consider what diagnoses were made on patients prior to the 1980s when Lyme Disease was first identified. How could future infection be reduced or prevented in endemic areas?

2. Review the literature on cutaneous infection and transplant recipients. What are the risk factors? What advice should transplant recipients be given about skin care? Should transplant recipients have regular dermatological reviews, and if you think this is necessary, what specific points would you include in your regular reviews?

Growth points

1. A new herpes virus associated with Kaposi's sarcoma

For some years, clinical observation has suggested that patients with AIDS who develop Kaposi's sarcoma may have a second infection in addition to HIV. Recent work by Chang and his colleagues has suggested that there is a previously unrecognized herpes virus involved. This has been called the Kaposi's associated herpes like virus—KSHV, and is found in a very high proportion of Kaposi's tissue. Work is in progress to establish the specificity of this observation, as preliminary reports suggest that the DNA footprints of this virus may be found in several other diseases.

2. Methicillin resistant staphylococci

Overuse and possibly inappropriate use of antistaphylococcal antibiotics has perhaps inevitably resulted in the development of strains of staphylococci resistant to conventional antistaphylococcal antibiotics. This has been seen in children with severe atopic dermatitis who have used large quantities of antibiotics such as mupirocin continuously for long periods. This is of concern to the wider hospital population as resistant staphylococci in emergency rooms and intensive care facilities result in major treatment problems for seriously ill patients with staphylococcal septicaemia. It is important therefore to use antistaphylococcal antibiotics thoughtfully and sensibly in managing patients with skin disease. In practice, the majority of these patients will have atopic eczema.

Further reading

Penneys, N. (1995). *Skin manifestations of AIDS* (2nd edn). Duntiz, London.

Canizares, O. and Harman, R. (ed.) (1992). *Clinical tropical dermatology*. Blackwell Scientific Publications, Oxford.

Parish, L.C., Witowski, J.A., and Vassileva, S. (1995). *Colour atlas of cutaneous infections*. Blackwell Scientific Publications, Oxford.

Autoimmune diseases and disorders of collagen and elastic tissue

- Lupus erythematosus: chronic discoid
  subacute cutaneous
  systemic
  neonatal

- Scleroderma: systemic sclerosis (generalized scleroderma, acrosclerosis)
  morphoea

- Lichen sclerosus et atrophicus (white spot disease)

- Dermatomyositis (polymyositis)

- Ehlers–Danlos syndrome (cutis hyperelastica)

- Pseudoxanthoma elasticum

Lupus erythematosus, scleroderma, and dermatomyositis are frequently referred to as collagen diseases but, as there is little specific association with collagen, autoimmune is a more appropriate description. This is because all are associated with a high incidence of circulating autoantibodies, some of which are of value in confirming a diagnosis. The term 'collagen' disease is appropriate for the Ehlers–Danlos group of disorders, as they are associated with genetically determined defects in the various types of collagen, and pseudoxanthoma elasticum is a disorder of elastic tissue.

Problem cases

Case 7.1

A 23-year-old female consults you about what she considers to be severe facial sunburn. She has just returned from her honeymoon on a Mediterranean island where she was exposed to strong sunshine , and three months earlier had started taking the oral contraceptive. On questioning she also complains of tiredness and joint pains. What conditions would you consider in the differential diagnosis, what investigations would you carry out, and what would be your management plan?

Case 7.2

A 70-year-old male comes to your consulting room complaining of severe tiredness and weakness. He also has a red macular rash running along the dorsa of his fingers and up the backs of his hands. What diagnosis does this description suggest, and how would you confirm it? What treatment would you prescribe, and are there any additional investigations which might be appropriate?

Lupus erythematosus

This is a spectrum of disorders, ranging from a relatively benign, purely cutaneous, localized problem to a severe and life threatening systemic disorder with minimal cutaneous involvement but severe and progressive damage to other organs such as the kidneys. In between these two extremes there are a number of presentations of intermediate severity such as subacute cutaneous lupus erythematosus, and patients may progress from one presentation to another in the course of their disease.

Table 7.1 lists the majority of the clinical presentations of lupus erythematosus with their usual associated autoantibody findings.

Table 7.1.

Clinical features of the main varieties of lupus erythematosus and rarer subsets, with commonly associated autoantibody findings

	Clinical features	Autoantibody profile
Systemic lupus erythematosus	Multisystem (renal, cardiac, CNS, etc.)	High-titre antinuclear antibody
	Facial photosensitivity and 'butterfly' erythema	Antibodies to double-stranded DNA
Chronic discoid lupus erythematosus	Photosensitive scaling and scarring lesions on light-exposed sites	Usually none
		In 5–10% low-titre antinuclear antibody
Subacute cutaneous lupus erythematosus	Extensive erythematous macules, usually on upper trunk and arms	Anti Ro and La in 20%
Chilblain lupus	Chilblain-like lesions on hands and feet	Usually none
Erythema multiforme-like lupus erythematosus (Rowell's syndrome)		Commonly anti-La
Neonatal lupus erythematosus	Facial erythema	Mother has circulating anti-Ro
	Complete heart block	
Systemic lupus erythematosus with thrombotic episodes and recurrent abortions	Livedo (prominent vascular) pattern in skin	Antiphospholipid antibodies
	CNS complications	

Pathology

The dermatopathological feature common to all types of lupus erythematosus is the lichenoid tissue reaction, a pattern seen also in other skin diseases. The term lichenoid tissue reaction is used when there is a vacuolar alteration of the basal cells in the epidermis, and an underlying lymphocytic infiltrate. There is usually also epidermal hyperkeratosis, and patchy thickening of the granular layer. This pattern is also seen in lichen planus (p. 62) and lichenoid drug reactions and, therefore, is not diagnostic of lupus erythematosus.

Immunopathology can also be helpful in confirming a diagnosis of lupus erythematosus. Direct immunofluorescence of clinically involved skin shows a course band of immunoglobulin, usually IgM or IgG in association with C3 at the dermo-epidermal junction. In patients with severe systemic LE, this immunoglobulin deposit may also be seen in clinically normal skin.

The presence and type of circulating autoantibodies is also used to make a diagnosis. In patients with purely cutaneous discoid lupus erythematosus, tests for circulating antinuclear antibodies of any type are usually negative, and only 5–10 per cent of patients have low titre (1:20–1:40) circulating autoantibodies. However, in those with more severe forms of subacute cutaneous LE and sys-

Key Points

Lupus erythematosus, scleroderma, and dermatomyositis are associated with autoantibodies, and these are of use in confirming diagnosis.

temic LE high titre circulating antinuclear autoantibodies (1:1000 or higher) are common. These may be directed against both double and single stranded DNA. In patients with subacute forms of LE anti-Ro (SSA) and anti-La (SSB) antibodies may also be present and are regarded as almost diagnostic. These antibodies are often not included in routine autoantibody screens, and must be specially requested from the laboratory if subacute LE is considered a possible diagnosis on clinical grounds.

Chronic discoid lupus erythematosus (CDLE)

Definition

A chronic, purely cutaneous disorder characterized by photosensitivity leading to the development of erythematous plaques on light exposed areas which heal with scarring.

Incidence and aetiology

Discoid LE is not a common dermatological disorder, but causes concern and referral out of proportion to its incidence because the face is the most commonly affected site, and because of permanent scarring which may be seen. Although the condition is triggered by sun exposure, the mechanisms involved are not yet understood. Females are more often affected than males.

Pathology

This is discussed above in the context of all types of lupus erythematosus. Biopsy shows a lichenoid tissue reaction which adds weight to the clinical diagnosis but does not confirm it as this pattern is not specific to CDLE.

Clinical features

CDLE usually begins in the sunny summer months as a tumid, raised, red, scaling plaques on the face (Figs 7.1 and 7.2). These scales are very adherent to the under-lying epidermis and run into the follicles, giving the so called carpet-tack sign. This means that when a scale is pulled off a plaque, there is an obvious little ex-tension on the underside which has come from an underlying pilosebaceous folli-cle opening. These plaques may be multiple and the scalp may be involved. The plaques slowly heal with scarring (Fig. 7.3) and on the scalp this will be associ-ated with areas of permanent alopecia, (Fig. 7.4) as the hair roots have been de-stroyed. There is no systemic upset. Over the winter months the problem usually becomes quiescent, but is reactivated in the next summer season.

Treatment

The use of a high SPF broad spectrum sunscreen by day will help prevent new lesions developing, and moderate to strong potent topical steroids will help reduce inflammation and scarring in lesions already present. CDLE is an

Figs 7.1 and 7.2 The facial appearance of two young girls with chronic discoid lupus ery-thematosus. Note the striking scaling involving the central panel of the face.

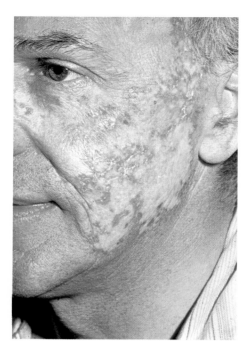

Fig. 7.3 Striking scarring on the face of a male with CDLE.

Fig. 7.4 Scalp involvement in chronic discoid lupus erythematosus. Note scarring and hair loss some of which will be permanent.

exception to the rule that strong topical steroids should not be used on the face, but even in CDLE regular review and steroid potency reduction is needed.

There is some evidence that the longer wavelengths of ultraviolet radiation are important in the pathogenesis of CDLE, and therefore sunscreens which offer protection well into the UVA range (320–360 nm) should be prescribed. Physical sunscreens such as microfine titanium dioxide are useful.

If in spite of a regime of sunscreens by day and topical steroids by night, new CDLE plaques continue to appear, systemic antimalarials should be considered. Chloroquine (maximum dose 150 mg/day) or hydroxychloroquine sulphate (Plaquenil, maximum dose 200 mg/day) can be helpful, usually given only over 4–6 summer months each year. Antimalarial drugs can cause cumulative toxicity in the eye, and it is therefore important to arrange for ophthalomolgical assessment prior to starting treatment if long-term use is envisaged. Cosmetic camouflage using Covermark or Dermablend may be very helpful to those with burnt out scarred lesions of CDLE on the face.

Subacute cutaneous lupus erythematosus (SCLE)

This variant of LE is part of the spectrum between purely cutaneous discoid LE, described above, and systemic LE.

Clinical features

Patients are photosensitive, and have red, macular lesions and also plaques on exposed skin (Fig. 7.5) but also on covered skin (Figs 7.6 and 7.7). The upper part of the trunk is often involved with diffuse and widespread lesions which persist throughout the year. Scaling and scarring are unusual.

The usual clinical differential diagnoses include other causes of photosensitivity such as polymorphic light eruption and photosensitive drug eruptions. Biopsy and immunofluorescence studies will be helpful, and the presence of circulating anti-Ro (SSA) antibodies in 60 per cent of patients and anti-La (SSB) in 40 per cent will all help confirm the diagnosis.

Treatment

These patients need topical sunscreens, and many respond well to systemic antimalarials as for CDLE. For patients with more persistent disease which continues throughout the winter months, a low dose of systemic steroids (for example prednisolone 10–20 mg/day) may be needed.

These patients are at risk of progression to multisystem SLE, and should therefore be monitored carefully.

There is also some evidence that those with a clinical pattern resembling either chilblains (Fig. 7.8), or an erythema multiforme like pattern are at greatest risk of disease progression.

Systemic lupus erythematosus (SLE)

Women are much more often affected than men.

Fig. 7.5 Subacute lupus erythematosus involving the cheek. Note raised tumourous relatively non-scaling lesions.

Figs 7.6 and 7.7 Lesions of subacute LE on the trunk. Note striking annular erythema in Fig. 7.7.

The classic SLE rash is a macular erythema over the face. While the cheeks and nose, the so-called 'butterfly area' are often heavily involved, the erythema may be rather more diffuse and generalized over the face (Fig. 7.9). This may be provoked by sun exposure. In addition, a variety of drugs, listed in Table 7.2, are known to induce SLE, sometimes in association with sunlight. The palms of the hands may show a diffuse erythema (Fig. 7.10), not unlike that seen in patients with liver disease, and the backs of the hands may show a diffuse mottled pattern, particularly after sun exposure.

Patchy, diffuse hair loss is a common feature but, as there is no scarring or permanent damage to the hair bulbs, the hair will regrow normally after successful treatment.

These patients frequently have symptoms related to other systems, such as joint pain, fatigue, breathlessness, ankle swelling, and polyuria. Consequently,

Fig. 7.8 Chilblain LE on the hands.

Fig. 7.9 The diffuse erythema of systemic lupus erythematosis.

Table 7.2.
Some of the commoner drugs known to induce an SLE-like syndrome or SLE

Hydralazine	INAH
Methyldopa	Phenylbutazone
Griseofulvin	Procaine amide
Oral contraceptives	Sulphonamides
Penicillin	Diphenylhydantoin

Fig. 7.10 The palms in SLE. Note the erythema and telangiectasia.

before they start treatment a detailed clinical and laboratory assessment is essential to establish the extent of disease involvement.

Investigations

More specialized investigations will depend on the systems thought, on the basis of history and clinical examination, to be involved in the disease process. Table 7.3 lists appropriate baseline investigations.

Diagnosis and treatment

In a patient who is obviously generally unwell and who has a butterfly rash provoked by sunlight, SLE is a likely diagnosis. Antinuclear antibody and DNA binding determination are the most useful confirmatory laboratory tests. A careful drug history should be taken to exclude drug-induced SLE. Occasionally, other photosensitive eruptions may mimic SLE, but in these cases there is no systemic upset and no anti-double-stranded DNA antibodies.

Treatment of SLE is usually based on systemic corticosteroids together with, in some cases, an immunosuppressive agent such as cyclophosphamide, azathio-prine, or chlorambucil as a steroid-sparing agent. The starting dose will depend on the patient's condition, but often a dose of 50–100 mg of prednisolone daily is required. It should be reduced as the patient's clinical condition improves. For monitoring disease activity DNA binding may be useful and a sudden rise may give warning of a relapse. Maintenance steroid therapy should be as low as

Table 7.3.
Investigations in suspected systemic lupus erythematosus

Essential

ESR and/or C reactive protein

Full blood count—Hb, WBC, platelets

Liver function tests

Urea, electrolytes, creatinine clearance

CXR

ECG

Urinalysis

ANA, anti-double-stranded DNA, C_3C_4, CH50 levels

Skin biopsy and immunopathology

Additional possible investigations

Renal biopsy

Pulmonary function

Lumbar puncture

EEG

possible to limit long-term side-effects, and alternate-day regimes are of value. The addition of immunosuppressives is also helpful in this respect and some patients can be maintained on these drugs alone. Whichever regime is found best for the individual patient, all require careful fortnightly or monthly supervision to monitor activation of disease and to screen for treatment-induced side-effects. Azathioprine, cyclophosphamide, and chlorambucil are most likely to produce haematological or renal toxicity, while hypertension, weight gain, glycosuria, and electrolyte imbalance are the principal hazards for the steroid-treated patient.

Topical therapy is a minor factor in managing these patients, although sun avoidance is important. A sun-screen with a sun protection factor (SPF) of 10 or more (For example Coppertone supershade 15, Roc 15) and a topical steroid by night may accelerate improvement of cutaneous lesions, even in patients receiving relatively high doses of systemic steroids.

Over the past decade the prognosis for patients with SLE has steadily improved, possibly due to earlier diagnosis and more effective treatment.

Neonatal lupus erythematosus

This is a rare LE variant but it is important to be aware of it if working with neonates. The affected child may have red, circular or arcuate lesions, usually on the face and upper trunk. The more serious problem is that virtually all these children have complete heart block, and neonatal LE is one of the commonest causes of this condition. The mother of the child will have circulating anti-Ro antibodies, and subsequent infants are also at risk.

SLE with thrombotic episodes

This variant of LE is associated with cerebrovascular accidents, myocardial infarction, other thrombotic episodes, and, in the case of females, a poor obstetric history with multiple miscarriages.

A common cutaneous finding is the so-called livedo pattern—a striking accentuation of the superficial vascular patterns on the skin, usually best seen on the thighs.

Affected patients have circulating antiphospholipid antibodies, which include the lupus anticoagulant, antibodies to cardiolipin, and to phosphatidylethanolamine.

Scleroderma

Scleroderma is the generic term for systemic sclerosis and morphoea. As with lupus erythematosus, there is a systemic form (systemic sclerosis) and a purely cutaneous or local form (morphoea).

Systemic sclerosis (generalized scleroderma, acrosclerosis)

Definition

A systemic disease characterized by progressive accumulation of collagen, fibrosis, and loss of mobility of the skin and other organs, such as the respiratory and gastrointestinal tracts. The kidneys may also be involved and in rare cases this is fulminating and leads rapidly to death.

Pathology

The striking feature seen in fully developed systemic sclerosis is a reduction of the normal thickness of the dermis for the body site biopsied. Thus, the subcutaneous fat is seen to be much closer to the epidermis than is normally the case. Endarteritis and minor inflammatory changes are found around blood vessels in the dermis. In contrast to morphoea, skin appendages are generally present in normal numbers.

Clinical features

Females are more commonly affected and many initially have severe Raynaud's phenomenon. The affected hands and feet are initially swollen and have tight, slightly atrophic skin which is bound firmly to the subcutaneous tissue (Fig. 7.11). The soft tissue of the mouth and palate are similarly affected, causing denture wearers to complain of poorly fitting plates because the mouth gradually shrinks. The face is often characteristic, with a strikingly line-free forehead, a small beaked nose, a small mouth with radial furrowing around the lips, and, in advanced cases, multiple dilated capillaries (telangiectasia) (Fig. 7.12 and 7.13). Small calcified nodules may develop in long-standing cases, usually in the skin of the hands and feet. A variant of this disorder has been named the CRST or

Fig. 7.11 The hand in progressive systemic sclerosis. Note the tightly bound skin, atrophy, and early gangrene in the middle finger.

CREST syndrome (c = calcification, R = Raynaud's disease, E = esophageal dysfunction, S = sclerodactyly, and T = telangiectasia) in which extensive multisystem involvement is said to be less common than in true systemic sclerosis.

Involvement of the gastrointestinal tract causes dysphagia and malabsorption through loss of peristalsis. Pulmonary involvement presents as dyspnoea and cardiovascular complications may lead to heart failure.

Laboratory findings

Most patients with progressive systemic sclerosis have high titres of circulating antinuclear antibody, usually of the speckled variety. Antiscleroderma-70 and anticentromere antibodies are also found in a high proportion of patients. On X-ray, the jaw in dentulous patients shows a widened peridontal membrane, and the hands may show resorption of the distal phalanges and early flecks of subcutaneous calcification. On barium swallow there is loss of oesophageal peristalsis.

Pulmonary function tests show impaired diffusion and serial renal function tests may show rapid renal failure, the most serious complication of this disorder.

Diagnosis and treatment

Diagnosis is often made clinically, simply on the appearance of the patient as she enters the clinic. Confirmatory tests include a skin biopsy, an autoantibody screen, hand and jaw X-ray, barium swallow, and respiratory function tests.

Treatment is largely symptomatic but, although there is little evidence that systemic steroids affect the course of this disease, they are certainly justified in patients with severe respiratory or renal involvement. The disease tends to progress slowly but, as some cases burn themselves out, it is difficult to assess the value of any therapeutic procedure. Hands and feet should be kept warm and regular professional chiropody offered. A trial of sympathetic blockade will indicate whether or not surgical sympathectomy is likely to be of value, but this is rarely the case.

Three groups of drugs may be of value in the management of Raynaud's disease or Raynaud's phenomenon complicating one of the collagen disorders, usually systemic sclerosis or lupus erythematosus. These are the prostacyclins, ketanserin, and nifedipine (Adalat). The prostacyclins have been shown in small-scale double-blind studies to raise the temperatures of the hands and fingers, and bring about pain relief in patients with Raynaud's phenomenon. The 5-hydroxytryptamine receptor antagonist, ketanserin, has also been used in double-blind studies in patients with both Raynaud's phenomenon and Raynaud's disease; significant improvement has been shown in both blood flow and skin temperature measurements. The dose required is 20 mg three times per day and no significant side-effects are recorded.

Nifedipine, the calcium channel blocker, has also been reported to be of value in patients with Raynaud's phenomenon and Raynaud's disease. As yet there is no reported trial comparing these three approaches in the management of Raynaud's disease.

Trials of intramuscular interferon have produced mixed results.

Figs 7.12 and 7.13 Facial appearance in progressive systemic sclerosis. Note loss of lines on forehead, relatively beaked nose, radial furring around the mouth, and telangiectasia.

Morphoea

Definition

A purely cutaneous disorder seen most commonly in children or young adults and characterized by the spontaneous appearance of a scar-like band or plaque on any body site.

Pathology

Loss of all skin appendages is the major feature in the histology of morphoea, giving a rather 'empty' look to the dermis. The collagen bundles are larger than usual and tend to run parallel to the skin surface. The normal difference between the papillary and reticular dermis is thus lost, and the overlying epidermis tends to be thin and atrophic.

Clinical features

Morphoea presents as a rather firm, white or violet patch of skin on any body site, commonly the thighs, trunk, and upper arms (Fig. 7.14). In any developing lesion there is a well-marked red or violet margin. As the disease activity burns out, this edge assumes the same colour as the central lesion and the white area becomes very firm with an atrophic, glazed epidermis. Calcification within the lesion is seen.

A linear variant of morphoea may occur, usually on the scalp and face (so-called '*en coup de sabre*'), and gives rise to alopecia and to growth irregularities of the underlying skull if in a young child. In morphoea post inflammatory melanin pigmentation tends to develop in 'burnt out' lesions.

Diagnosis and treatment

The clinical appearance is commonly diagnostic and biopsy is rarely required. In very early lesions, when erythema rather than a firm white atrophic plaque is

Fig. 7.14 Ivory white patch of morphea. On palpation this will be firm and indurated with a rather plaque-like feel.

seen, the lesion may have to be observed for 2–3 months before a firm diagnosis can be made. Biopsy at this stage is not always helpful as the fully developed histological picture is not present.

At present there is no specific treatment. Topical steroids or intralesional corticosteroid injections into an active lesion may alter its final shape, but will not arrest its development.

Lichen sclerosus et atrophicus (LSA) ('white spot disease')

Definition

An atrophic condition, commonly of the vulva, sometimes associated with morphoea on other body sites.

LSA and morphoea are found together more frequently than can be attributed to chance. White, atrophic, glazed areas of skin with follicular plugging develop (Fig. 7.15), and may progress to extreme atrophy and shrinkage of genital tissue. The lesions may ulcerate and cause pain and pruritus, although some are asymptomatic. LSA usually affects the female genitalia. It rarely affects the penis in the male, when it is called balanitis xerotica obliterans. Extragenital lesions are most common around the neck and upper back. There is a reported incidence of 1–4 per cent of malignant change in vulvar LSA. This has not been reported with prepubertal LSA which usually clears spontaneously at puberty.

Children with LSA frequently complain of genital discomfort and bleeding. A number of such children have been inappropriately suspected of being victims of child sexual abuse. It is obviously important to be aware of childhood LSA and to ensure that those in other professions, such as social work, are also aware of its existence so that such potentially serious mistakes are avoided.

Fig. 7.15 Lichen sclerosus et atrophicus of the shoulder area. Note the atrophic white macules. Vulvar lesions are very commonly seen in patients with these extragenital lesions.

Diagnosis and treatment

Diagnosis is usually made clinically although biopsy may be required in atypical cases.

Treatment is unsatisfactory and unnecessary for asymptomatic lesions. Pruritus and ulceration are helped by topical steroid preparations (for example vioform hydrocortisone cream) or topical oestrogens (for example Dinoestrol cream).

Long-term follow-up is required in all severe cases as malignancy may not supervene until the lesion has been present for 20 years or more.

Dermatomyositis (polymyositis)

Definition

A disorder of skin and muscle characterized by a specific skin rash and muscle weakness.

Dermatomyositis is relatively rare. There are two varieties, one affecting children, the other adults.

Pathology

The cutaneous lesions show histological changes similar to those seen in SLE. Liquefaction degeneration of the basal layer is common, and the overlying epidermis may be thin and atrophic. In the dermis, large numbers of free melanin granules are seen due to pigmentary incontinence. Free red cells are also present, the result of capillary leakage.

The degree of muscle involvement is variable but, if affected, the muscle shows fibre degeneration and internalization of the sarcolemmal nuclei.

Clinical features

The typical rash of dermatomyositis is a macular erythema on the face, particularly marked in the periorbital area where it is described as heliotrope or blue violet (Fig. 7.16). The dorsa of the hands and fingers are also involved with linear erythema and nodules (Gottron's papules) (Figs 7.17 and 7.18). Nail-fold haemorrhages may also be seen, but these are common to all the connective tissue disorders. Erythema can also appear on the neck and upper chest, and progress to poikiloderma (dappled skin) which consists of telangiectasia alternating with atrophy. Photosensitivity is common.

Muscle weakness is very variable. It most commonly affects the proximal muscle groups of all four limbs, so that early weakness tends to be noted on climbing stairs or performing tasks with the hands at or above shoulder level. It may become very severe, and respiratory difficulties can result from involvement of intercostal and diaphragmatic muscles.

In childhood, dermatomyositis tends to 'burn out', but may leave severe restriction of limb movement due to calcification in and around muscles.

Fig. 7.16 Facial appearance of a patient with dermatomyositis showing characteristic violet discoloration around the eyes.

Figs 7.17 and 7.18 The hands of an Indian patient with dermatomyositis. Note erythema on the backs of the fingers and Gottrens papules on the sides.

Diagnosis and treatment

Diagnosis is usually based on the combination of a typical skin rash, muscle weakness, and raised circulating muscle enzymes (SGOT, SGPT, creatine kinase, and aldolase). If muscle biopsy is to be performed, electromyography will indicate a suitable area of involved muscle.

There is continuing unresolved controversy over the association between dermatomyositis and detection of a previously occult malignancy. Current evidence suggests that in at least some series this is a significant association in older individuals, but that the malignancy will be detected by a good routine medical assessment, and that extreme measures such as laparotomy are not justified in a hunt for such a malignancy. Common sites for such a malignancy include the gastrointestinal tract, the prostate, the ovaries, and the breast.

Removal of a malignancy if present may result in spontaneous, although usually temporary, improvement of the muscle weakness. If no malignancy is found, systemic steroid therapy may give symptomatic relief and a trial of prednisolone 20–60 mg/day is justified. Systemic azathioprine (150 mg/day) may also be of value either alone or as a steroid-sparing measure. Disease activity should be monitored by regular assays of muscle enzyme levels.

Ehlers–Danlos syndrome (cutis hyperelastica)

Definition

A group of inherited disorders characterized by defects in dermal collagen.

At the present time eleven biochemical variants of this true 'collagen' disorder are recognized. Modes of inheritance are both autosomal dominant and sex-linked recessive. The basic defects in collagen synthesis are both quantitative and qualitative, and can be accurately identified by fibroblast culture and biochemical assay. On light microscopy the collagen appears whorled and disorganized, and in some cases there is an associated increase in elastic fibres. Type 4 EDS is associated with a defect in type 3 collagen and type 5 in a deficiency in the enzyme lysyl hydroxylase. In the other variants, the exact biochemical problem has not yet been identified.

Clinical features

Clinically, the skin is hyperelastic (Fig. 7.19), fragile, and bruises easily. The joints have lax capsules, are hyperextensible, and readily undergo subluxation. Poor posture and hernia formation may, in part, be due to muscular hypotonia. Poor healing of minor skin trauma leaves ugly scars (Fig. 7.20 and 7.21). The patients have striking blue sclerae. In some cases the collagen of large vessels is also affected,

Fig. 7.19 Striking cutis hyperelastica of the Ehlers–Danlos syndrome.

Figs 7.20 and 7.21 Poorly formed scars over the ankle and knee area in patient with Ehlers–Danlos syndrome.

and death due to dissecting aneurysm or spontaneous vessel rupture is recorded. A proportion of patients also have features of pseudoxanthoma elasticum.

Diagnosis and treatment

Diagnosis is based on the clinical appearance and a positive family history, and should be confirmed by biochemical studies on fibroblast cultures. No treatment is yet available, but identification of the type of Ehlers–Danlos will aid genetic counselling.

Pseudoxanthoma elasticum

Definition

A hereditary disorder of elastic tissue.

Like the Ehlers–Danlos syndrome, the are genetically distinct variants. Both autosomal dominant and autosomal recessive varieties are recognized. At present, genes coding for elastin and fibrillin are considered likely candidates.

Pathology

The characteristic pathological feature is the presence in the dermis of tangled, degenerate elastic fibres on which calcification readily occurs. This abnormality is also found in elastic tissue of the blood vessels and the heart.

Clinical features

The cutaneous lesions are found in the axillae and groins and are soft, yellowish papules—'chamois leather' skin (Figs 7.22, 7.23 and 7.24). Ocular lesions are common and can be seen on ophthalmoscopy as angioid streaks, haemorrhage,

Figs 7.22, 7.23 and 7.24 Features of the skin of the flexure areas in pseudoxanthoma elasticum.

and choroiditis. Some degree of visual impairment is common. Involvement of major blood vessels may give rise to hypertension, angina, and haemorrhage including haematemesis.

Diagnosis and treatment

Diagnosis is based on the clinical appearance, a positive family history, and the histology. No specific therapy is available.

Discussion of problem cases

Case 7.1

The differential diagnosis here includes a range of photosensitive disorders such as polymorphic light eruption, a photosensitive drug eruption, and lupus erythematosus. The history of systemic upset suggests that polymorphic light eruption is unlikely, but both SLE and photosensitive drug eruptions can cause generalized problems. As all the cutaneous erythema was on the face, and mainly on the central panel, a biopsy was not carried out initially. On examination, the patient had a blood pressure of 180/120 mm Hg and electrolyte and liver function tests showed a markedly elevated serum urea and creatinine. She also had high titre circulating autoantibodies to double stranded DNA. This last result confirms a diagnosis of systemic lupus erythematosus, possibly precipitated in a genetically predisposed individual by exogenous oestrogens in the oral contraceptive, and by sun exposure.

The patient was started on high doses of oral steroids (prednisolone 80 mg/day), and the oral contraceptive withdrawn. Over the next four weeks her blood pressure fell and her urea and creatinine returned to the normal range. Her facial erythema slowly cleared without scarring, and the dose of oral steroid was reduced to 15 mg on alternate days 3 months after her first presentation.

What is her prognosis? What other organs are at risk? She wishes to start a family and asks you if there are any risks to herself during pregnancy or to the baby. How will you reply?

Case 7.2

This male patient has muscle weakness and a rash. The likely diagnosis is therefore dermatomyositis. Investigations which will help confirm this diagnosis are electromyography (EMG), levels of circulating muscle enzymes in the peripheral blood, and muscle biopsy.

The patient had circulating creatine phosphokinase levels of over 20 times the upper limit of the normal range. This was considered adequate to confirm the diagnosis, and the patient was given oral prednisolone 100 mg/day. There was a very rapid response with increase in muscle power. Because of the possibility of his dermatomyositis being associated with an occult malignancy a CT scan of the thorax abdomen and pelvis was carried out and the levels of prostate specific antigen measured. No abnormalities were found, and over a period of 14 weeks his prednisolone level was reduced to 20 mg/day. What will be your ongoing management plan for this patient?

Projects

1. There have been suggestions that dermatological conditions other than Lyme disease (described in Chapter 6) are caused by *Borrelia burgdorferi*. These include morphoea and lichen sclerosus et atrophicus. Run an appropriate literature search, and make the case both for and against such an association.

2. Review the literature on the genetics of the various types of Ehlers–Danlos syndrome and the severity of the clinical phenotype associated with each. Draw up a list of points you would consider important to discuss with young adults in each of the genotypes who wished genetic counselling.

3. Make a comprehensive list of all the dermatological problems which might be responsible for presenting to his or her doctor with a red face, and draw up a programme of investigation which would allow you to make an accurate diagnosis in every case.

Growth points

Dermatology and the new genetics

At present, dermatology is making a considerable contribution to the new genetics. It is likely that over the next few years the genes associated with Ehlers–Danlos and pseudoxanthoma elasticum variants will be identified. These are both good examples of groups of disease where there are clear metabolic markers. In the case of lupus erythematosus there is obviously a much more complex interaction between genetic susceptibility and environmental provoking factors, but even here it is possible that a number of LE susceptibility genes will be identified.

Further reading

Wallace, D.J. and Hannahs Hahn, B. (1992) *Dubous lupus erythematosus* (4th edn). Lea and Feibiger, Philadelphia and London.

Royce, P.M. and Steinmann, B. (eds) (1993). *Connective tissue and its heritable disorders*. Wiley-Liss, Chichester.

8

Disorders of the vasculature

- Vascular naevi: Haemangiomas
  Salmon patches
  Vascular malformations

- Leg ulcers—   venous and arterial

- Vasculitis: Erythema nodosum
  Pityriasis lichenoides
  Polyarteritis nodosa
  Cutaneous polyarteritis
  Lupus pernio
  Lupus erythematosus
  Allergic vasculitis
  Giant cell arteritis

- Pyoderma gangrenosum

- Temporal arteritis

- Erythema induratum

- Urticaria

- Henoch–Schoenlein purpura

Problem cases

Case 8.1

A 62-year-old obese retired school teacher consults you because of a small leg ulcer at her right ankle. She has been treating it herself with over the counter remedies and a cream given to her by her sister. The skin around the ulcer is very red and inflamed. What is your investigation and management plan?

Case 8.2

A 23-year-old male consults you about the regular appearance of what he describes as red weals on his skin. These have been appearing over the past 6 months and his face is usually involved. What is the likely diagnosis and what investigations and treatment will you suggest?

Case 8.3

Both parents come to see you with their first child, a girl now aged 6 months. She has a red, raised mark covering about 10 per cent of her forehead. The parents are very agitated as they have been told elsewhere that no treatment is needed, but the mark is still expanding. They want to know about laser treatment and why their child is being denied this therapy. What is the diagnosis and what will you tell them about therapy?

Disorders of the arteries, veins, and capillaries may all present with skin problems. Some are predominantly cutaneous disorders affecting only the cutaneous vasculature, and others are more generalized, involving many systems, the skin included. In young children, the most common problem is that of vascular naevi, and in older adults the most frequent presentation is with lower leg ulceration which may be due to either venous or arterial malfunction. Capillary disorders often cause a purpuric eruption and vasculitis can produce painful nodular ulcerating lesions. Vascular pathology is most commonly seen on the lower legs as their circulation is subject to stasis. Biopsies from the lower leg have to be interpreted with care in older adults, as histology of clinically normal skin of this area may show minor vascular changes due to gravity.

Vascular naevi

Vascular naevi are seen in a very high proportion of young babies. The three subsets of vascular naevi are:

Key Points

A very high proportion of babies have vascular naevi but most forms fade spontaneously.

Fig. 8.1 Mixed, predominantly cavernous angioma. Child is 3 months old.

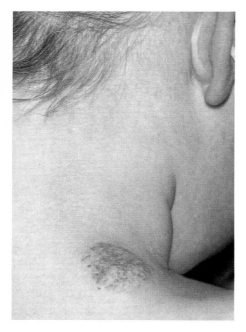

Fig. 8.2 The child in Fig. 8.1 aged 3 years, to demonstrate spontaneous resolution. Further improvement can confidently be expected.

- haemangiomas
- salmon patches
- vascular malformations.

Haemangiomas

Definition

Benign proliferations of the vascular endothelium.

About one child in ten develops a cutaneous angioma during the first month of life. They are not usually apparent at birth. The commonest type is the strawberry mark or cavernous haemangioma, which usually expands rapidly during the first year of life, then slowly and spontaneously shrinks over the next 3–4 years (Figs 8.1 and 8.2), so that by the time the child is ready for school there may be some loose redundant skin. Occasionally they are very large indeed, and there may be concern about either haemorrhage or obstruction of vision leading to blindness in the affected eye.

Treatment

As the great majority of strawberry haemangiomas shrink spontaneously, and this results in minimal long-term scarring, parents should be told of this, and encouraged to let this happen. Showing sequential photographs of older patients whose lesions have cleared spontaneously will be helpful. Bleeding which may occur should be controlled with firm pressure, and infection, if the lesion becomes ulcerated, treated with an appropriate topical antibiotic. Both bleeding and infection appear to accelerate spontaneous resolution.

The **deep cavernous angioma** has all the features described for the superficial cavernous angioma, but in addition there appears to be a proliferation of vessels in the deeper capillary plexus. These do not shrink as completely as the superficial vessels, and resolution is usually less complete.

Rarely, with the giant lesions, treatment with either systemic steroids or intralesional injections of either steroids or interferon may be necessary. For this group of angiomas, there is little evidence, at present, that laser therapy gives a better long-term result than natural involution, and the main concern of the doctor involved should be to select the treatment option that will result in least long-term scarring when the child is a teenager and adult. Minor plastic surgery may be needed for the larger lesion to remove folds of redundant skin when natural shrinkage is completed.

Rare variants of cavernous angiomata can be associated with systemic abnormalities, such as thrombocytopenic purpura, and any infant who has a very large lesion or with a family history of angiomata should be appropriately investigated.

Salmon patches (telangiectatic naevi, Unnas naevus, stork bite)

These faint macular lesions are seen in as many as a third of all new-born infants. They are usually on the nape of the neck or the central panel of the face. They are composed of distended and persisting fetal dermal capillaries. The majority fade spontaneously in the first few months of life, but those on the nape of the neck may persist. This is not usually a problem.

Vascular malformations (naevus flammeus, port wine stain)

Definition

A persisting macular area of erythema due to dilated superficial capillaries.

These lesions are present at birth, and the majority affect the facial skin over the area served by the trigeminal nerve. Initially they are deep red and macular. Here there is no tendency for spontaneous resolution, and raised nodules may develop on the naevus as the child grows. Very large port wine stains may be associated with additional vascular abnormalities of the cerebral vessels giving rise to the Sturge–Weber Syndrome.

Treatment

This can be either by cosmetic camouflage or by laser destruction of the abnormal vessels. Pulsed, tuneable dye lasers give best results with least scarring, and are becoming available in many centres. Usually several treatments are equired, and sedation of a young child will be needed to maintain the head absolutely still. Results are excellent, and current policy is to try to offer laser therapy early in life before the naevus has become raised and palpable. Clearly, there are at present a number of adults in the community for whom laser treatment was not an option when they were young. Results in these more mature naevi are less satisfactory, and camouflage therapy using Dermablend or Cover mark preparations may be more appropriate. In the UK, the Red Cross run an excellent cosmetic camouflage advisory and demonstration service (Figs 8.3–8.6).

Figs 8.3, 8.4, 8.5, and 8.6 Port wine stains before and after application of camouflage cover.

Leg ulceration

Seventy to eighty per cent of ulcers on the lower legs result from venous damage, due to the increased venous pressure associated with varicose veins and past venous thrombosis. The remaining 20–30 per cent result from arterial damage. It is important to understand the basic principles of leg ulcer management, and even more important to recognize patients at risk of developing an ulcer in the first place and offer advice to help prevent this happening. The main at risk group for venous leg ulcers are obese females with varicose veins, who may have had past problems with venous thrombosis, perhaps during pregnancy.

Venous leg ulcers (stasis ulcers, gravitational ulcers)

Incidence and pathological features

Venous ulceration is very common in Britain and accounts for around 3 per cent of all new cases attending dermatological clinics. The incidence in the community is much higher as many patients either attend their general practitioner or seek no medical assistance. Most patients are women.

Venous leg ulcers develop because of incompetent valves in the leg veins. There is secondary increase in capillary pressure, with stasis, capillary damage, fibrosis, and a poorly nourished skin which is easily damaged by minor trauma.

Clinical features

The typical patient is an obese, middle-aged woman. A past history of a deep venous thrombosis is common and varicose veins are usually present. One or both legs may be involved (Fig. 8.7). The most common site of ulceration is over the medial malleolus, and the surrounding skin frequently shows gross fibrosis,

Key Points

Most ulcers on the lower leg result from venous damage.

Fig. 8.7 Venous stasis ulceration. Note typical site over medial malleolus and trophic changes in surrounding skin.

purpura, and livedo due to extravasation of blood from damaged capillaries, an appearance termed '**atrophie blanche**'. The ulcer is frequently precipitated by minor local trauma. Stasis ulcers are commonly single and although they may be extremely large they are relatively pain-free, in contrast to arterial ulcers. The surrounding skin is frequently oedematous, eczematous, and secondarily infected.

Arterial leg ulcers are much less common and usually develop as a complication of a general vasculitic problem such as systemic lupus erythematosus or rheumatoid arthritis. They are usually multiple, extremely painful, and are seen over the whole calf, not just around the ankle.

Diagnosis

The diagnosis of a leg ulcer is self-evident. It is necessary to establish, however, whether the lesion is of purely vascular origin or whether it is part of a generalized disease and, if vascular, whether it is due to arterial or venous disease. This can be done easily by using the Doppler non-invasive ultrasound technique to detect direction of flow in vessels, and establish whether or not underlying valves in veins are competent.

Treatment

Treatment of an established venous leg ulcer consists not only of symptomatic therapy designed to promote healing but also of prophylaxis to reduce the risk of recurrence. These measures include surgical treatment of varicose veins, weight reduction, and the use of supportive elastic stockings and protective bandaging.

The basic principles of management of an established venous leg ulcer are the maintenance of a clean, healthy ulcer base free of infection, and protection of the surrounding skin to allow re-epithelialization to take place. Unfortunately, this is easier to write than to practise as the damage resulting in the leg ulcer has usually built up over decades. The base of the ulcer is frequently a poor surface for new epidermis and, even if healing can be achieved, breakdown of the healed area after minor trauma is all too common.

A variety of astringent preparations will help to maintain a clean healthy ulcer base. These include 20 per cent benzoyl peroxide (Benoxyl) and sodium hypochlorite 1 in 4 (Milton solution). Topical antibiotics should not be used routinely on clinically clean ulcer bases. For very moist exudative ulcers 2–3 days treatment with absorbent dextranomer beads (Debrisan) will assist in drying the lesions, but this preparation should not be continued for long periods. If the ulcer is obviously infected, swabs should be sent for bacteriological sensitivities and the infection then treated with an appropriate antibiotic.

Occlusive dressings have been shown in experimental studies to provide a more physiological environment to allow the ulcer to heal. Although expensive, they are worth using and a wide range are available (for example Geliperm. Granuflex, Tegasorb, Sorbsan). These usually have a gel or colloid formulation which absorbs exudate from the ulcer and thus accelerates re-epithelialization. They are also extremely comfortable for the patient and usually bring about almost instant pain relief. If the ulcer is not producing a lot of exudate, they can be left in position for up to 7 days.

Key Points

> The aim of treating a venous leg ulcer is to prevent infection and allow healing.

The skin surrounding the actual ulcer may be erythematous and irritable with a stasis dermatitis reaction. While this is often responsive to topical steroid preparations, they must be used with caution in this situation and kept away from the ulcer base otherwise they will delay healing. They should not be used constantly on the skin around the ulcer as they will, in time, cause atrophy and possibly further extension of the ulcer. For this reason the surrounding skin is best protected with a waterproof paste such as plain zinc paste BP or zinc paste with salicylic acid (Lassar's Paste).

Adhesive bandages such as Viscopaste or Ichthopaste are also helpful, particularly for patients who have persistent stasis dermatitis around the ulcer area. Four layer bandaging using an absorbent crepe next to the dressing, followed by padded support (for example velband), followed by a firm bandage of the blue line type, followed by a final coband bandage is extremely effective and comfortable for patients with proven venous ulcers. These four layers are available as a Profore pack (Smith and Nephew).

Patients, their carers, and district or practice nurses should all be given a demonstration of how to apply these bandages. Once the ulcer is healed, patients should use an elastic stocking of appropriate grade to try to prevent recurrence.

Patients with chronic leg ulcers are at risk of developing an allergic contact dermatitis to medicaments. Patch testing to medicaments should be considered if there is persistent inflammation around the ulcer area.

In severe cases resistant to treatment outlined above, pinch grafting may be considered. Although this gives good initial results, there is a high recurrence rate once the patient is ambulant.

Remember that redness and inflammation around the leg ulcer may be an allergic contact dermatitis to a prescribed medicament. If in doubt, patch test.

Arterial leg ulcers

Patients with arterial leg ulcers present with severe pain. This may be particularly intense on elevating the legs and may interfere with sleep. These ulcers are considerably less common than the venous variety and affect both sexes equally.

In a typical case, the patient has no evidence of varicose veins, but has poor peripheral pulses and multiple small painful ulcers, which have a punched-out appearance and are situated in the lower third of the leg (Fig. 8.8). As arterial leg ulcers are frequently associated with generalized arterial pathology, it is important to look for diabetes, atherosclerosis, Buerger's disease, and rheumatoid arthritis.

Diagnosis and treatment

Pain and the site of the lesion may help to differentiate an arterial from a venous ulcer, and further useful pointers are the absence of varicose veins or of a history of deep venous thrombosis.

Systemic diseases associated with vascular ulcers include diabetes mellitus, syphilis, lesions of the spinal cord, rheumatoid arthritis, and polyarteritis nodosa. Sickle cell disease and other haemoglobinopathies must be considered in patients of Mediterranean origin. In a long-standing leg ulcer with atypical features the possibility of malignant change should be borne in mind and biopsy performed.

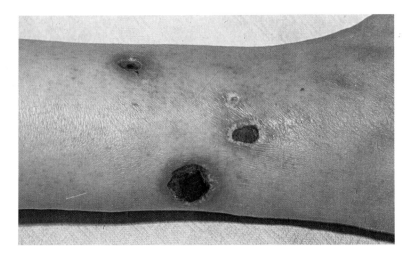

Treatment is mainly symptomatic. Topical therapy as for venous ulcers is useful but pressure bandaging is not appropriate. Rest and warmth are of particular importance. Systemic vasodilators may give symptomatic relief in a few cases, but it is debatable whether this is more than a placebo effect. Sympathectomy may be of value and a trial nerve block should be performed to determine whether or not relief of pain can be achieved.

Vasculitis

Definition

A pathological process centred primarily on blood vessel walls (mainly small- and medium-sized vessels) resulting in purpura, nodules, and ulceration.

Pathology

The classification of vasculitis is confusing, and can be based either on clinical or on pathological features. Table 8.1 is based on the pathology and relies on the predominant cell type seen around the damaged vessel.

It is crucial in the histological diagnosis of vasculitis to see unequivocal damage to the vessel wall as many conditions are associated with a perivascular cellular infiltrate, but no frank damage to the vessel. Even a classification of this type is unsatisfactory, as it is likely that different cell populations will be seen within a lesion at different stages of its development.

Clinical presentations of lymphocytic vasculitis

Erythema nodosum

Definition

A lymphocytic vasculitis seen mainly in women (F:M = 5:1) and predominantly affecting the lower legs.

Table 8.1.

The main types of vasculitis classified according to predominant cell type in the infiltrate

Predominant cell type	Clinical conditions
Lymphocyte	Chilbains (lupus pernio)
	Lupus erythematosus
	Erythema nodosum
	Pityriasis lichenoides
Polymorph	Polyarteritis nodosa
	Allergic vasculitis
	Henoch–Schoenlein purpura
Granuloma formation	Giant cell arteritis
	Erythema induratum

Clinical features

Erythema nodosum is characterized by painful, palpable, dusky blue-red lesions on the calves and shins, although occasionally the forearms are also affected. General malaise, fever, and joint pains are common. The lesions slowly resolve over a period of 2–4 weeks. At this stage the gradual fading of the lesions has an appearance very similar to simple bruises (Fig. 8.9).

Fig. 8.9 Erythema nodosum. The lesions can be very faint, but are indurated and painful on palpation.

Erythema nodosum is an example of a tissue reaction and may be caused by a variety of problems. The current commonest causes in the UK are adverse drug reactions, streptococcal infection, sarcoidosis, viral and chlamydial infections, and tuberculosis. In other European countries *Yersinia* infection is a relatively common precipitating factor. However, in the majority of cases no clear cause is identified.

Table 8.2 outlines a reasonable, appropriate plan of investigation for cases of erythema nodosum.

Table 8.2.
Investigation plan for erythema nodosum

1	History, including a careful drug history
2	E.S.R.
3	Throat swab, ASO titre
4	Chest X-ray (sarcoid, tuberculosis
5	Mantoux test (*before* Kveim test)
6	If Mantoux test negative, Kveim test
7	Viral titres, both acute and convalescent

The clinical picture of a febrile patient with painful, non-ulcerating leg nodules is diagnostic. Treatment is mainly symptomatic. If the condition is thought to be drug-induced, the suspected drug should be withdrawn. Bed rest, elevation of the limb, and systemic analgesics should be prescribed. The value of topical preparations is debatable, but 10 per cent ichthyol in water applied twice daily to acute lesions is a comfort to some patients. Steroids topically are of no value, and there is little evidence that, given systemically, they change the course of the disease.

Pityriasis lichenoides acuta

Definition
A purely cutaneous disorder of unknown aetiology characterized by multiple papules and plaques.

Pathology
Histopathologically, there is a lymphocytic vasculitis.

Clinical features
Pityriasis lichenoides acuta presents as multiple, pruritic, excoriated papules, occurring in crops on the trunk and limbs. Purpuric lesions are occasionally seen.

There is rarely any systemic upset, and spontaneous remission is usual but may take months or years to occur.

Diagnosis and treatment

Diagnosis is based on the clinical appearance and is usually confirmed by biopsy. Insect bites and atypical dermatitis herpetiformis are the most common causes of confusion, but the possibility of the papular form of secondary syphilis should be borne in mind. Syphilitic lesions will commonly affect the palms and soles, whereas those of pityriasis lichenoides will only do so rarely.

Treatment is usually based on moderate potency topical steroids. A course of ultraviolet light will benefit some patients.

Clinical presentation of polymorphonuclear vasculitis

Polyarteritis nodosa

Definition

A rare, severe, generalized disease characterized by necrotizing arteritis.

Pathology

Histologically, there are polymorphonuclear leucocytes in the blood vessel walls and fragments of disintegrating nuclei from damaged polymorphs ('nuclear dust') will be seen.

Clinical features

The patient is generally unwell and may be febrile. Subcutaneous nodules, subungual splinter haemorrhages, small purpuric lesions, and, occasionally, frankly gangrenous lesions may be present. As this is a multisystem disorder, other signs and symptoms result from involvement of the renal, abdominal, cardiovascular, and CNS vasculature (Fig. 8.10).

Key Points

Always take a careful drug history in a patient with erythema nodosum.

Fig. 8.10 Necrotizing (leucocytoclastic) vasculitis. Palpable lesions are surrounded by purpura and tend to break down easily.

Occasionally a milder variant is seen which appears to be confined to the skin and consists of a livedo pattern on the skin of the lower legs, associated with leg nodules. This has been called **cutaneous polyarteritis nodosa.**

Diagnosis and treatment

Diagnosis is based on evidence of involvement of multiple vessels and is usually confirmed by biopsy. Treatment with systemic steroids and immunosuppressives (for example azathioprine) is required, but even so there is a significant mortality.

For patients with the cutaneous variant, low doses of systemic steroids may also be needed. Simple analgesics such as aspirin will relieve pain. Topical steroid therapy is of little value.

Pyoderma gangrenosum

Definition

A rare dermatological disorder in which large, ulcerating lesions appear suddenly and dramatically.

Pathology

Pyoderma gangrenosum results from underlying thrombosis and vasculitis.

Clinical features

The initial cutaneous lesions resemble indolent boils, but they rapidly expand, break down, and leave large, ulcerated, painful areas. Systemic upset, with fever and malaise, is frequent. Pyoderma gangrenosum may be the first signs of ulcerative colitis, Crohn's disease, rheumatoid arthritis, and monoclonal gammopathies or frank myeloma (Fig. 8.11).

Fig. 8.11 Pyoderma gangrenosum. These large lesions can develop with dramatic rapidity.

Diagnosis and treatment

The diagnosis is generally apparent on clinical grounds. Systemic steroid therapy should be prescribed in a moderately high dose (for example 60–100 mg of prednisolone daily) and subsequently reduced as the lesions heal. If there is only one lesion, intralesional injection of steroid may be helpful, provided it is injected into an early lesion. A soothing non-adherent dressing should be applied (for example Scherisorb).

Clinical conditions associated with granulomatous vasculitis

Temporal arteritis (giant cell arteritis)

Definition

A rapidly progressive granulomatous arteritis which can cause blindness if not recognized and treated promptly.

Clinical features

The classic presentation of temporal arteritis is that of an elderly person complaining of severe headache and general malaise, often with some associated visual upset. There may be red palpable nodules in the temporal area.

These patients usually have a very high erythrocyte sedimentation rate, and a temporal biopsy should be performed as a matter of urgency to confirm the diagnosis. Systemic steroids in high doses should be started without waiting for the pathology report as there is a real risk of blindness.

Erythema induratum (Bazin's disease)

A condition affecting the lower legs of young women, currently believed to be a hypersensitivity reaction to the tubercle bacillus.

This condition is relatively rare and presents as painful ulcerating nodules on the back of the lower legs of obese patients, usually female.

Treatment is difficult, but weight reduction and keeping the legs warm in appropriate trousers or tights are worthwhile. A long-term trial of full anti-tuberculous therapy should be considered, but there are no controlled comparative studies proving the value of antituberculous therapy.

Urticaria

Definition

Recurrent, transient, cutaneous swellings and erythema due to fluid transfer from the vasculature to the dermis.

This condition is common and varies from minor but inconvenient cutaneous lesions to the severe life-threatening angio-oedema affecting the

Key Points

Urticarial lesions around the mouth is an emergency condition and patients should be observed for signs of respiratory obstruction. Subcutaneous adrenaline may be required.

laryngeal area. A local sudden increase in capillary permeability is the common final pathway for a variety of stimuli thought to cause urticaria.

Some of the recognized types of urticaria are listed below. The majority of cases will fall into the group of unknown aetiology.

The urticarial lesion is a rapidly developing raised weal or plaque (Fig. 8.12). Lesions may be large, multiple, and appear with alarming speed. Lesions occurring around the mouth should be regarded as a dermatological emergency, and the patient observed for signs of respiratory obstruction. Many patients have a chronic variety of urticaria, resistant to therapy, which persists for months or years before burning out.

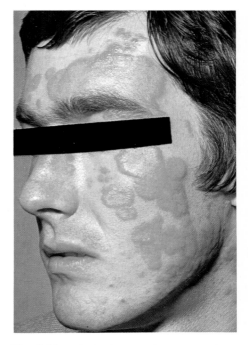

Fig. 8.12 Urticaria. Large erythematous weals are seen on the face.

Recognized varieties of urticaria

1. **Due to histamine-liberating drugs**. Salicylates are the commonest group of drugs in this category and patients with chronic urticaria should be advised to use paracetamol rather than aspirin as a simple analgesic. Codeine, morphine, and indomethacin will also release histamine and should, therefore, be avoided.
2. **Due to ingested food additives**. The two food additives known to cause or provoke urticaria are the tartrazine group of dyes, found in yellow- and orange-coloured drinks and sweets, and benzoates, used widely as preservatives.
3. **Contact urticaria**. Here the lesions develop only on actual sites of contact, for example on the site of contact with dog hair or saliva, or on the lips after ingesting protein foods. This variety of urticaria is common in atopic patients.
4. **Physical urticaria**. In a small group of patients pressure, heat, cold, and sunlight may provoke urticarial weals.
5. **Urticaria and hereditary angio-oedema**. This rare condition is transmitted by autosomal dominant inheritance. The basic biochemical defect is in the complement pathway. The enzyme C_1 esterase inhibitor is lacking in these patients who may present with gross and alarming swellings. They may also present as acute surgical emergencies because of sudden oedema of a part of the small intestine leading to acute pain and obstruction.
6. **Related to general medical problems**. This is a miscellaneous group. Patients infested with parasites tend to develop urticaria, as do those with chronic bacterial infection in such sites as the nasal sinuses and the urinary tract. Patients with lupus erythematosus, thyrotoxicosis, and lymphomata may also present with urticaria.
7. **No known or identifiable causative factor**. This comprises by far the largest group of patients.

Diagnosis and treatment

Diagnosis is self-evident and patients frequently do not seek help until they have tried several home remedies. These should be identified in case they are histamine releasing agents.

The investigation of a case of urticaria can be a time-consuming, expensive, and non-rewarding exercise and, as the disease is common, a sensible compromise is to investigate only patients who have had recurrent attacks for 6–9 months duration or longer who do not obtain relief from systemic antihistamine therapy. Patients

Table 8.3.

An outline of investigations for cases of chronic persistent urticaria

Full blood count (Hb, WBC+ eosinophil count, platelets)

Liver function tests

Chest and sinus X-ray

Examination of hot stool for parasites

Examination of urine for bacteria

Complement screen including C_1 esterase inhibitor

Autoantibody screen

should be told that tests will rarely reveal the cause of the urticaria, and that in time the problem will resolve spontaneously. A reasonable battery of investigations to be performed as an out-patient is detailed in Table 8.3. A careful history should identify the rare cases of physical urticaria and may be a pointer in cases provoked by food additives. The great majority of cases will yield negative results on this screen and must be treated on a symptomatic basis.

Treatment of acute urticaria may require subcutaneous adrenalin as a life-saving measure. For chronic cases the cornerstone of therapy are systemic H1 antihistamines and often several need to be tried before one is found which combines symptomatic relief with minimal side-effects. Current popular, non-sedating antihistamines include cetirizine (Zirtek), loratadine (Clarytin) terfenadine (Triludan), and astemizole (Hismanal). All are relatively non-sedating. While there is little published evidence that the addition of an H2 inhibitor adds to the effect of the H1 inhibitor, it may be worth adding cimetidine in adequate doses in severe and persistent urticaria. A moderate potency topical steroid may be useful for symptomatic relief of established lesions.

For more persistent cases, the possibility of elimination diets should be considered and patients should be advised about avoiding tartrazine and benzoate containing food and drink. More specific dietary elimination treatment requires expert supervision from a dietician, particularly if provocation tests with the suspected foodstuff is part of the plan.

Systemic steroids are not appropriate for chronic urticaria, but a short 5–7 day course may be necessary for acute and widespread urticaria.

Purpura

Purpura may be caused by a platelet disorder, a disease affecting capillaries, or a more general systematized disease. Common causes of purpura are ageing (in which the small blood vessels of the skin lose their normal collagen support), topical or systemic steroid therapy (which similarly increases capillary fragility), vitamin C deficiency, and side-effects of drug therapy. Rarer causes include generalized amyloidosis and renal disease. Platelet counts of 60 000/mm^3 or more are unlikely to produce purpura and, in patients with platelet counts above this level, causes of non-thrombocytopenic purpura should be sought.

Henoch–Schoenlein purpura (anaphylactoid purpura)

Definition

A purpuric eruption due in some cases to an allergic reaction to bacteria, systemic drugs, associated with fever, malaise, and gastrointestinal and renal involvement.

Pathology

The underlying pathological lesion is a vasculitis affecting small vessels and the degree of systemic involvement is very variable. Children are frequently affected.

Clinical features

Macular or papular purpuric lesions are scattered on the limbs and buttocks. General malaise and fever may be present, as may arthralgia, haematuria, and abdominal pain. The platelet count is normal. In some patients there is a history of a streptococcal throat infection 7–14 days prior to development of purpura, and in others there is a history of systemic drug ingestion. In most cases, however, no cause can be identified.

Diagnosis and treatment

Diagnosis is usually straightforward and investigations should be carried out to establish the degree of systemic involvement. The most serious complication is severe renal involvement which can lead to the nephrotic syndrome. The disease is usually self-limiting and there is little evidence that systemic steroids will alter its course. Nevertheless, they are frequently prescribed for patients with severe multisystem involvement. Bed rest and simple analgesics may be required for arthropathy. Urinalysis should be performed and repeated to look for frank haematuria and developing proteinuria.

Discussion of problem cases

Case 8.1

The history and the patient strongly suggests that this is a venous leg ulcer rather than an arterial ulcer. The contributing factors include the female sex, obesity, and a history of a job which involves standing for long periods of time.

This can be confirmed by the fact that the arteries around the ankle have good pulses and Doppler ultrasound confirming the fact that the valves in the perforating veins in her legs are incompetent.

In the history it emerged that she had been treating the ulcer with a moderately potent steroid. This was withdrawn and an occlusive dressing applied to the ulcer with a weak potency steroid (1 per cent hydrocortisone) around the ulcer. On this regime there continued to be a lot of inflammation and irritation. Patch testing was, therefore, arranged to establish whether or not any of the medicaments the lady was using was contributing to her problem. The patch test battery included the topical corticosteroid tixocortol, and she was shown to have a topical steroid allergy. All topical steroid was, therefore, withdrawn and copious emollients and occlusive dressings applied under four layer bandaging. On this regime the ulcer healed in 10 weeks. During this time she was encouraged to try to lose some weight, and once the ulcer was healed she was referred for consideration for surgery to her varicose veins.

Case 8.2

The diagnosis here strongly suggests urticaria. This has been persistent but has not caused any general debility, and the patient has lost no time from work.

A careful history has established that from time-to-time this patient does take aspirin for minor aches and pains. He was, therefore, warned against the use of aspirin and other histamine releasing drugs. A full history revealed no other possible causes of his urticaria. A blood count showed no evidence of eosinophilia. He was, therefore, started on a regime of H1 antihistamines, and returned at 3 weekly intervals to report progress. On the third non-sedating antihistamine his urticaria improved significantly with only two minor episodes each week. These disappeared completely over the next few months.

This history illustrates the fact that most patients with urticaria have a self limiting condition which burns out after a period of 6 months to a year. Extensive investigations very rarely uncover the trigger for urticaria, and are expensive and time consuming for the patient.

Case 8.3

The history is that of a cavernous angioma, a vascular naevus associated with proliferation of the capillary endothelial cells. These are very common, but as they tend to grow through the first year of life, they do cause concern particularly as many of them are on the face. Many patients have read in the newspapers of the significant advances made using laser treatment for a variety of other vascular lesions, and are concerned that their child is not getting state of the art treatment. At the present time laser treatment is not the most appropriate method of managing a cavernous angioma or strawberry naevus, as natural regression of the lesion will usually produce the best result.

This was explained to the parents, and photographs of older children whose lesions had regressed spontaneously were shown to encourage them. They were also given the address of the Naevus Support Group to put them in contact with other parents in the same situation. The parents departed reassured that their child was not being denied essential treatment. Eighteen months later there had been very significant reduction in the size of the lesion, and by the time the child was three the lesion was virtually invisible.

Projects

1. Look in MIMS, the British National Formulary, or the Physicians Desk Query (PDQ) for currently available occlusive dressings. Look at the cost of these and the size of the packs in which they are supplied. Work out a table for the best buys of these assuming you are treating three patients all of whom have leg ulcers 6 cm in diameter over a period of 5 months. Work out a rough estimate of the cost of materials for treating these ulcers taking into account both occlusive dressings and bandaging.

2. Find out if your hospital or health centre has standing orders or guidelines for the management of acute anaphylaxis. This can begin with severe urticaria, so the dermatology service should be aware of their existence. If they are available, review them with colleagues. If none appear to exist, draw up draft guidelines as to when you would use adrenaline and systemic steroids and how you would protect the airway.

Growth point

The use of cultured keratinocytes as a dressing for chronic ulcers

Routine culture of normal human keratinocytes is now possible and one can take a skin biopsy from an area of normal epidermis, grow the keratinocytes on a suitable substrate, and then, usually after about 6 weeks growth *in vitro*, layer this sheet of keratinocytes on to a leg ulcer as a graft. This has been carried out both with the patient's own cultured keratinocytes, and also with cells from an unrelated donor. In both cases healing is accelerated. This may be due to the presence of epidermal growth factors in the cells. The allogeneic non-self cells do not take but form a useful dressing for a short period.

Further reading

Falanga, V. and Eaglestein, W. (1995). *Leg and foot ulcers, a clinicians guide*. Martin Dunitz, London.

Disorders of the cutaneous melanocyte

- Freckles (lentigines)

- Actinic lentigines

- Melanocytic naevi—banal, Spitz, halo, congenital, atypical, and blue

- Albinism

- Vitiligo

- Chloasma

- Addison's disease

The structure and melanin-producing function of the epidermal melanocyte network has already been described (p. 16). The evolutionary function of epidermal melanocytes is considered to have been the production of a protective pigment layer in response to exposure to sunlight as a protection against damaging wavelengths of solar radiation.

The commonest abnormalities in the distribution, structure, and function of melanocytes with the resulting clinical condition are listed in Table 9.1. All, with the exception of malignant melanoma, are discussed in this chapter.

Problem cases

Case 9.1

A 38-year-old, fair skinned, auburn haired woman comes to consult you about two irregular macules, on her shoulder. She was born in South Africa and lived in that country until she came to the UK as a student. She has large numbers of freckles and also large numbers of naevi, mainly on her trunk and limbs. She misses the warm South African sunshine and uses a sunbed regularly at home. What investigations will you carry out on the two lesions on her shoulder which are both about a centimetre in diameter and irregular in outline? What advice will you offer her in general?

Case 9.2

An Asian student at the local technical college consults you about patchy depigmentation on her trunk. She is reluctant to undress completely, but the lesions are asymptomatic and you make a diagnosis of vitiligo. You tell her there is little that can be done. She returns 3 months later to tell you that the depigmented areas are now itchy, and that her two younger sisters have developed the same problem. What action do you take?

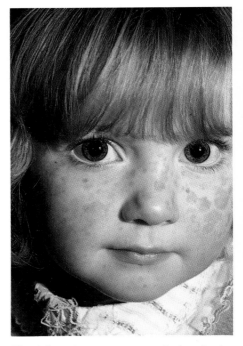

Fig. 9.1 Freckles or lentigines on the face of a young girl.

Freckles (lentigines)

Freckles or lentigines are simple areas of overactivity of an increased number of melanocytes which are confined to the basal layer of the epidermis (Fig. 9.1). They are found in large numbers in fair or red haired individuals of Celtic descent. Their development is stimulated by sun exposure in genetically predisposed individuals. Their importance lies in the fact that they are a marker of an individual with relatively sun sensitive skin who should receive advice about rationing sun exposure.

Table 9.1.

Melanocyte abnormalities and their clinical manifestations

Melanocyte abnormality	Clinical manifestation
Generalized non-function of melanocytes	Albinism
Localized loss of melanocytes	Vitiligo
Localized increase in melanogenesis	Freckles (ephelides)
Hormonally-mediated increase in melanogenesis	Chloasma
Localized increase in numbers of epidermal and dermal melanocytes	Junctional and compound naevi
Localized increase in numbers of dermal melanocytes	Mongolian spot, blue naevus, naevus of Ota, naevus of Ito
Localized increase in both epidermal and dermal melanocytes and naevus cells	Giant pigmented hairy naevus
Malignant change in epidermal melanocytes	Malignant melanoma

Actinic lentigines (PUVA or UVA freckles)

These are large (1 cm diameter or more), macular, brown lesions which develop in individuals who have received a lot of UVA from sun beds or in the course of PUVA therapy. They are also seen on the sun exposed skin of older people, and even in young adults after severe sunburn. The shoulders are a common site for this (Fig. 9.2).

Melanocytic naevi (moles)

Pigmented melanocytic naevi or moles are extremely common and at present a very common cause for specialist referral, mainly because of concern that they might be early malignant melanoma (p. 294). The majority of naevi first appear on the skin during the second decade of life, and the average young white-skinned adult has 20–50 such naevi. With age, many of these naevi disappear spontaneously.

There are two current points of importance concerning banal melanocytic naevi:

1. It is important to be able to distinguish common banal naevi from early melanoma.

Key Points

The presence of a large number of melanocytic naevi is a risk factor for melanoma.

Fig. 9.2 Actinic lentisos following sunburn on the shoulder of a young boy.

2. The presence of larger than average numbers of small naevi is a risk factor for melanoma, not necessarily arising on a naevus, but at any site on the body surface. Patients with large numbers of banal naevi should, therefore, receive advice on reducing sun exposure, and should be taught to recognize and seek medical help for lesions which may be early, curable malignant melanoma.

The commonest clinical types of pigmented naevi are:

- banal acquired naevi—by far the largest group;

- halo naevi;

- Spitz naevi;

- congenital naevi, including the rare but important giant garment or bathing trunk naevus;

- clinically atypical naevi (dysplastic naevi), either familial or sporadic;

- blue naevi, arising from dermal melanocytes.

Pathology

The majority of melanocytic naevi arise from the basal layer melanocytes and are junctional, compound, or intradermal (Fig. 9.3). Junctional means that all the benign, proliferating melanocyte or naevus cells, which comprise the naevus, are in contact with the overlying epidermis; compound means that there are, in addition, small clusters of naevus cells lying free in the underlying epidermis; and intradermal means that all the naevus cells are lying in the dermis in small clusters under a completely normal epidermis.

Banal or acquired melanocytic naevi

These lesions are very common. They are small (usually 2–3 mm in diameter) and a uniform brown (Fig. 9.4). In younger patients these naevi are a pale brown

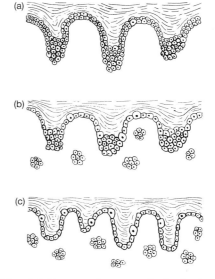

Fig. 9.3 Patterns of naevus cell distribution in melanocytic naevi. (a) Junctional naevus; (b) compound naevus; (c) intradermal naevus.

Fig. 9.4 Compound naevus on the neck of a young woman. The lesion is a uniform brown, slightly raised, and about 4 mm in the largest diameter.

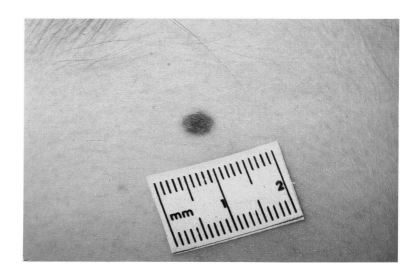

but as the patient, and the naevus, matures it frequently becomes darker, and may become elevated. With further ageing, many of these naevi, particularly on the face, lose their pigment completely and appear as flesh-coloured skin tags (Fig. 9.5), often with an outgrowth of one or two terminal hairs.

Banal melanocytic naevi should only be excised if they have changed in shape, size, or colour, or if there are any other grounds for concern about malignant change. The chances of malignant change in any one naevus are very small indeed, and there is no place for extensive preventive excision. If a naevus is excised, always send it for pathological examination.

Fig. 9.5 Intradermal naevus on the face of a 45-year-old woman. Note the lack of pigment, the visible capillaries, and terminal hair growth.

Halo naevi

These are common and harmless. They are usually compound naevi with a halo of surrounding depigmentation. They are frequently seen on the backs of teenagers during the summer months, and are much more easily seen on darker skin than on pale skin (Figs 9.6 and 9.7). Over the next few months, the central naevus will disappear, leaving a pale area which may take years to repigment. While this is happening, the area should be protected from strong sunlight as there are no melanocytes present and severe burning can occur.

Excision is not necessary.

Fig. 9.6 Halo naevi on coloured skin, note very striking depigmentation.

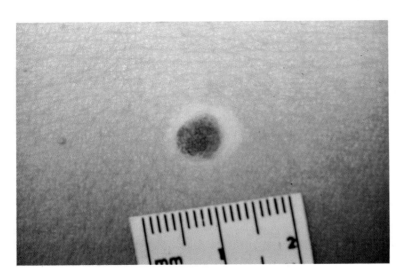

Fig. 9.7 Halo naevus on Caucasian skin, note much less dramatic appearance.

Spitz naevi (formerly called juvenile melanoma)

These naevi are most commonly seen on the faces of children but can occur at any age. They are variants of compound naevi and their importance lies in the fact that if excised they can be difficult for the pathologist to distinguish from malignant melanoma without a clear history of the age of the patient and the clinical appearance of the lesion. They usually present as a growing, pink or pale brown lesion on the cheek (Fig. 9.8) in a child but may be darker and more worrying in an adult.

Excision is rarely required in children but may be necessary in adults to rule out developing melanoma.

Fig. 9.9 Relatively small congential naevus on the face of a young girl.

Congenital melanocytic naevi

These are usually defined by size as small, medium, or giant. One per cent of all new-born babies have a small, congenital, pigmented melanocytic naevus. This is usually small (less than 5 cm in diameter; Fig. 9.9) and only pale brown at birth, although it may darken with time and also develop an outgrowth of terminal hair. The pathology of these lesions usually shows naevus cells infiltrating into the skin appendages in a manner not seen in the banal acquired naevi.

The giant congenital naevus (bathing trunk or garment naevus) is fortunately extremely rare (Fig. 9.10). This is a very large naevus usually covering a large part of the trunk, and sometimes also associated with several smaller congenital naevi. There is an increased life-time risk of malignant change in these giant naevi, and this may occur either in the cutaneous component or in the associated involvement frequently found in the central nervous system. For this reason early and complete removal of giant pigmented naevi is theoretically ideal, but in practice the surface area involved makes this very difficult.

Children born with a giant congenital melanocytic naevus should be referred to a local specialist in this field with no delay. Some authorities believe that the lesions should be dermabraded within the first week of life to reduce the naevus cell load, but long-term results of this approach are not yet available. An alternative or complementary approach is to use the techniques of tissue expansion by inserting inflatable balloons under normal skin to expand the normal skin and so create redundant epidermis which can then be used for definitive excision and grafting procedures. Obviously, neither of these procedures reduces the risk of malignant change outwith the skin.

Clinically atypical naevi

These melanocytic naevi are defined as naevi which are larger than banal naevi (> 4 mm in diameter), and have in addition at least one of an irregular edge, irregular colour, or inflammation. The pathological appearances may be described as dysplastic, a term which is poorly defined. Their importance is that larger numbers of such naevi are found on the skin of melanoma patients than would be expected by chance, so individuals with four or more of these naevi should also receive advice about rationing sun exposure and recognizing early melanoma.

Atypical naevi are found on all body sites, but are commoner on the male back and the female leg (Figs 9.11, 9.12, and 9.13).

Many atypical naevi have clinical features which make them difficult to distinguish from early malignant melanoma, and excision with a narrow margin of surrounding normal epidermis is therefore necessary. Some patients have large numbers of such naevi, and large scale excision is not practical. These patients should be referred to specialist centres who will manage them with a mixture of photography, regular review, and excision of any changing lesions.

Fig. 9.10 Giant pigmented hairy naevus. These lesions are also termed bathing trunk or garment naevi. There is a significant incidence of development of malignant melanoma in this type of lesion.

Figs 9.11 and 9.12 Clinically atypical naevi on the back of young males showing striking increase in normal numbers of naevi and in their size.

Fig. 9.13 Close up of a clinically atypical naevus showing irregular outline and irregular pigmentation.

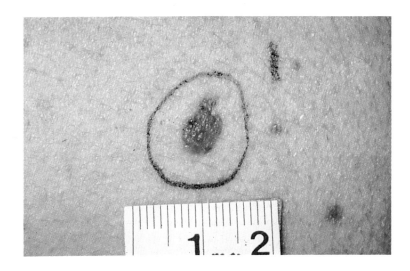

Blue naevi

These naevi arise from dermal melanocytes. They are usually first identified in late childhood as deep-blue or black lesions, commonly on the face, hands, or feet (Fig. 9.14). A variant of the blue naevus is seen on the sacral area of dark-skinned babies as the so-called Mongolian spot.

Blue naevi are frequently excised both for cosmetic reasons and also to rule out melanoma.

Fig. 9.14 Blue naevus on the nostril.

Key Points

In albinism the melanocytes either lack tyrosinase or have poor enzyme function.

Albinism

Definition

An autosomal recessive disorder, characterized by a lack of pigment production by melanocytes in the epidermis, hair bulb, and eye.

Pathology

The melanocyte either lacks tyrosinase necessary for melanin pigment synthesis (tyrosinase negative albinism) or has tyrosinase present but poorly functional (tyrosinase positive). These two varieties of albinism can be differentiated by incubating plucked hair bulbs *in vitro* with tyrosine or DOPA. The hair bulbs with functionally normal tyrosinase will show a black deposit, but in those without the enzyme there will be no pigment deposit. The tyrosinase gene is on chromosome 11, and allelic variants have been identified.

Clinical features

Lack of normal pigmentation is the striking feature of albinism. The skin is white or pink, the hair pale blonde, and the iris translucent. Sunlight is very poorly tolerated, and sunburn and photophobia are common symptoms. Nystagmus may also be present. Albinism is very striking in Negroes and, when exposed to tropical or subtropical sunlight, their skin ages prematurely and they have a high incidence of malignant skin tumours, mainly squamous carcinoma. In temperate climates, as in the UK, the presenting features are usually ocular.

Diagnosis and treatment

Diagnosis is straightforward and the biochemical type of oculocutaneous albinism can be established by hair bulb incubation (see above).

Prevention of sun damage is essential. Sun avoidance should be practised and where sunlight exposure is inevitable a sun-screen preparation with a sun protection factor (SPF) of 15 or more should be used. Regular clinical review is essential for early diagnosis of skin tumours. Ocular problems require specialist ophthalmological supervision.

Vitiligo

Definition

An area of acquired cutaneous depigmentation due to loss of normal melanocytes.

Vitiligo affects around 0.4 per cent of the European population, and prevalence figures for genetically dark-skinned races suggest that it is commoner among them. As has been discussed in Chapter 1, it is currently one of the commoner conditions referred for specialist dermatological assessment. A high proportion of affected patients have a positive family history.

There is a significant association with autoimmune diseases such as pernicious anaemia, thyroid disease, and Addison's disease, and antimelanocyte antibodies can be detected in a proportion of vitiligo patients suggesting that autoimmune destruction of melanocytes may be involved in the pathogenesis.

Key Points

Vitiligo appears to be hereditary and is associated with other autoimmune diseases.

Pathology

Dopa or silver staining techniques show that epidermal melanocytes are lost from the basal layer of the epidermis.

Clinical features

Patients present with slowly extending acquired loss of normal melanin pigment on any body site (Fig. 9.15 and 9.16). In white skinned individuals this can be of little cosmetic or medical concern but the appearance can be very unacceptable on exposed areas of darker skinned individuals. Vitiligo demonstrates the Koebner phenomenon as it is provoked by minor trauma.

The prognosis for vitiligo is very varied. In some individuals only a small area of skin is affected, and some spontaneous repigmentation occurs, but in others there is continuing and extensive loss. This can cause great distress, particularly if the affected areas are mainly exposed sites and the patient is dark skinned.

Diagnosis and treatment

Diagnosis is usually self-evident, but in coloured skin pityriasis versicolor can be confusing, so scrapings should be taken for mycological examination. Leprosy is a very much rarer possibility, but can worry the patient greatly. However, in leprosy the hypopigmented macules are usually anaesthetic. In cases of doubt a biopsy should be performed.

Treatment is unsatisfactory. Some patients achieve a reasonable cosmetic result with topical artificial tanning creams containing dihydroxyacetone, but those with a dark skin rarely find these preparations satisfactory. In some cases potent topical steroids may prevent further depigmentation and possibly even be associated with repigmentation. Photochemotherapy (psoralens + UVA = PUVA) is of some value in a very small proportion of patients, but is time-consuming and may carry long-term hazards. Grafting of autologous melanocytes, after taking a small biopsy from pigmented skin of the patient and expanding the melanocytes in tissue

Key Points

Cloasma is a hormonally stimulated increase in melanogenesis.

Fig. 9.15 Vitiligo. The areas in which melanin pigment has been lost are particularly prone to sunburn.

culture, can be effective for small areas but is time consuming, not always success-ful, and only available in a limited number of centres.

Patients must be warned that the affected skin is easily sunburned and that they should use a topical sunscreen.

The Vitiligo Society is a very active patient support group which raises funds for research and runs useful conferences. Many patients with vitiligo find mem-bership useful.

Remember that patients from dark-skinned races with vitiligo may be very concerned about leprosy which also causes loss of pigment. Be aware of this and offer reassurance.

Chloasma

Definition

A hormonally-stimulated increase in melanogenesis which mainly affects the face, and which is seen in pregnant women and those on the contraceptive pill.

Both oestrogens and progesterone can affect melanogenesis and cause in preg-nancy a mask-like increase in facial melanin pigment—chloasma uterinum (Fig. 9.17). This is commonest in females with naturally dark colouring and may take months to resolve after parturition. A similar appearance is seen in some women on oral contraception. Sunlight increases the depth of pigmentation. Circulating levels of melanocyte stimulating hormone are normal.

While most women find that the pigmentation clears after delivery, it can persist in some cases. These women should be advised that the oral contraceptive will aggravate the situation, and warned that the problem will almost certainly recur in future pregnancies. A high SPF sunscreen should be used.

Discussion of problem cases

Case 9.1

This description indicates that this patient is genetically disposed to actinic damage because of her hair colour, fair skin, and freckles. This has been com-pounded by her upbringing in a country where exposure to strong sunlight for long periods of the year is virtually unavoidable.

The possibilities, therefore, are that the two brown lesions on her shoulder area are actinic lentigos, or even frank, early skin cancer, probably of the melanocytic type.

Biopsies showed that both lesion were actinic lentigos, and in the report the pathologist commented, without being given a full history, on the severe actinic damage seen in the dermal collagen surrounding the lesions.

The two lesions for which she sought help have therefore been removed, but she also needs advice on reducing further actinic damage. The first step is to strongly recommend that she give up sunbed sessions. Sunbeds mainly emit UVA or long

Fig. 9.16 Vitiligo appearing on coloured skin. Note very striking depigmentation.

Fig. 9.17 Chloasma. This is seen both in pregnancy and in some users of the oral contraceptive pill. It can persist for some time after parturition or discontinuing the pill.

wave ultraviolet radiation (320–360 nm), and this contributes significantly to age changes of photoageing. Sunbeds may also contribute to skin cancer risk.

Early childhood natural sun exposure, as has been experienced by this patient, also contributes to the risk of both melanoma and non-melanoma skin cancer (see Chapter 13). This patient should, therefore, be advised to avoid excessive natural ultraviolet exposure, and be given a leaflet illustrating the features of early skin cancers of all types—melanoma, basal cell carcinoma, and squamous cell carcinoma—with advice to seek medical help if she notices any similar changes on her own skin. She also should be advised to avoid noon-day sun, and use a high SPF broad spectrum sunscreen in sunny weather.

Case 9.2

Vitiligo is relatively common in the Asian population, and would be a reasonable initial diagnosis. There is a genetic component to vitiligo, so more than one family member may well be involved. However, rapid onset of pruritic depigmentation in three family members almost simultaneously does not suggest vitiligo. These girls must be examined properly. This was done by a female doctor at their request, when it became clear that the pattern of depigmentation suggested pityriasis versicolor (p. 132) rather than vitiligo. Pityriasis versicolor is frequently slightly pruritic. Scrapings were taken from all three girls for mycological examination, and these confirmed the presence of *M. Furfur*, the causative organism of pityriasis versicolor. All three patients were treated with a topical imidazole cream with relief of symptoms and slow repigmentation.

Further reading

Ortonne, J.P., Mosher, J.B., and Fitzpatrick, T.B. (1983). *Vitiligo and other hypomelanoses of the hair and skin*. Plenum Publishing Co, New York.

10

Disorders of the skin appendages

- Disorders of the pilosebaceous follicle:
  Acne vulgaris
  Rosacea
  Perioral dermatitis

- Excessive loss of hair:
  Alopecia areata
  Androgenic alopecia—male pattern baldness
  Telogen effluvium
  Miscellaneous causes of hair loss—syphilis, systemic lupus erythematosus, endocrine disorder, nutrition, drugs, hair shaft defects, trichotillomania, naevoid abnormalities, fungal infection, chronic discoid lupus erythematosus, lichen planus, traction

- Excessive growth of hair:
  Hirsutism
  Hypertrichosis

- Disorders of the nails:
  Congenital nail disorders—nail-patella syndrome, pachy-onychia con genita
  Acquired nail disorders—Beau's lines, koilonychia, finger clubbing, paronychia, herpetic whitlow, paronychial tumours, iatrogenic nail disorders

- Disorders of the sweat glands:
  Eccrine gland disorders—miliaria, hyperhidrosis
  Apocrine gland disorder—hidradenitis suppurativa

Problem cases

Case 10.1

A female in her late twenties consults you about papules on her face. She has a job which involves meeting the public and finds the development of these lesions distressing and unacceptable. She is on no regular medication other than the oral contraceptive, and thinks herself that the problem is due to an allergy to makeup. She tells you that until this point in time she has always had an exceptionally good skin. What is the likely diagnosis, and what are the appropriate investigations and management plans for this patient?

Case 10.2

The mother of an 8-year-old boy who lives on a farm consults you about her son's recent hair loss. The boy has striking loss of hair, mainly on the crown in regular, circular areas. The underlying scalp looks healthy. What condition does this description suggest, and what is the differential diagnosis? What treatment would you recommend? What factors might affect the prognosis?

Case 10.3

A colleague asks your advice on the diagnosis and management of a male in his late twenties who has recurrent abcesses in both axillae. These began about 10 years ago and have persisted ever since. Several courses of systemic antibiotics have had little effect. Your colleague is concerned about the possibility that the patient has an immunodeficiency problem. What is the likely diagnosis and what treatments might be of value?

Disorders of the pilosebaceous follicle

Acne vulgaris

Definition

A disorder of the pilosebaceous follicles causing comedones (blackheads), papules, and pustules on the face, chest, and upper back.

Epidemiology and aetiology

Mild acne vulgaris is almost universal at some time during the second decade. Surveys of teenage school children suggest that girls develop acne 2–3 years earlier than boys, but that boys have rather more persistent lesions. Most acne

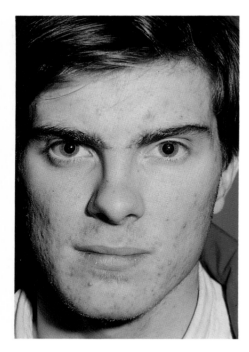

Fig. 10.1 Relatively mild acne vulgaris.

Fig. 10.2 More severe acne vulgaris, involving the cheeks and chin.

sufferers have a very mild form of the disease which can be managed with proprietary preparations, but a small proportion require help from their general practitioner and an even smaller group require specialist referral. There appears to be a growing number of older patients, usually women, in the third decade who have mild but stubborn acne persisting for over 10 years.

The four factors which contribute to development of the acne lesion are:

1. production of excessive sebaceous gland secretion;
2. obstruction to outflow of this sebum at the mouth of the pilosebaceous canal;
3. inflammation arising as a result of leakage of contents of the pilosebaceous follicle into the surrounding dermis;
4. excessive colonization or infection of the pilosebaceous ducts with *P. acnes*.

Sebaceous gland secretion is partly controlled by androgen stimulation. In the neonate small visible sebaceous glands are often seen on the central panel of the face due to stimulation by maternal androgens. After the first few days of life, these become vestigial until puberty when the individual's own androgen levels rise, causing expansion of the sebaceous glands and in many cases temporary overproduction of sebum.

Pathology

Classical acne is not normally biopsied. The picture is that of a distended pilosebaceous follicle with a surrounding cellular infiltrate in the dermis. If there has been rupture of the duct with leakage of its contents into the surrounding dermis, granuloma formation, foreign body giant cells, granulation tissue, and scar formation may also be seen.

Clinical features of classical acne vulgaris

The early lesions are open and closed comedones (blackheads and whiteheads), which develop into papules and pustules, mainly on the forehead, nose, and chin (Figs 10.1–10.5). In more severe cases the entire face with the exception of the periorbital skin may be affected, often with additional involvement of the upper chest and back. These sites are most densely populated with well developed sebaceous glands. Generally, acne is associated with clinical signs of excessive sebaceous secretion and a greasy facial skin and scalp. This interrelationship is not, however, exclusive because in other conditions (notably Parkinson's disease) associated with excessive sebaceous secretion there are no accompanying acne lesions. Many females with acne notice premenstrual deterioration of their lesions. If acne has been severe and persisted for some time leading to rupture of pilosebaceous follicles, there may be scarring. With modern methods of treating acne, this should be prevented by prompt treatment.

Variants

Tropical acne affects young Caucasians in a hot, humid environment such as the Far East. They develop gross acne lesions, mainly on the trunk, which can be disabling and resistant to all therapy other than return to a temperate climate.

Steroid acne appears in some patients on systemic steroid therapy. This acneiform eruption tends to affect the trunk rather more than the face and, although papules and pustules are present, comedones are notably absent.

Chemical acne is due to cutting oils and chlorinated hydrocarbons. This acneiform eruption is usually seen in those who handle these substances at work. They develop some lesions on atypical sites, such as the legs, due to protracted contact with oil in saturated working clothes.

Chloracne, a very disfiguring disorder, is fortunately rare, but the leakage of dioxin gas at the Seveso chemical plant brought publicity and recognition. Dioxin and chlorinated hydrocarbons are absorbed in the body, and cause an acneiform eruption, characterized by large numbers of occluded whiteheads (Fig. 10.6) and inflamed cysts. These may persist for very many months after only transient exposure.

Infantile acne is a rare variant in which acne lesions are seen in male infants, usually between the age of 3 and 12 months. If severe, endocrine studies should be undertaken to exclude an androgen-secreting lesion. There is some evidence that infants affected with acne are prone to develop severe lesions in the teenage years.

Fig. 10.3 Severe pustular acne vulgaris. This young man already has scarring.

Differential diagnosis

The clinical diagnosis of acne is usually simple, and is normally made by the patient prior to seeking advice. Acneiform drug eruptions should be considered, particularly in any patient presenting outwith the normal age range. Antituberculous and anti-epileptic drugs are both responsible not only for aggravating pre-existing acne, but also for provoking an acneiform eruption. Rosacea may give rise to confusion, but generally it is seen in an older age group. Although pustules may be present, there are no comedones and there is associated erythema.

Therapy

Acne therapy can be divided into topical therapy which may be all that is needed for mild acne, systemic therapy (including oral antibiotics and anti-androgens) which are needed for most acne patients referred for specialist opinion, and oral retinoids for patients with severe persistent acne who have not responded to first line systemic treatment.

Topical treatment for acne includes:

- benzoyl peroxide-containing preparations;

- topical antibiotics—erythromycin and tetracycline;

- topical vitamin A acid—tretinoin;

- antiseptics and keratolytics;

- azaleic acid preparations—Skinoren

- abrasive pastes.

Fig. 10.4 Acne vulgaris in an Indian showing extensive involvement in the face.

Fig. 10.5 Acne vulgaris of the back showing typical distribution.

Fig. 10.6 Chloracne of the side of the face showing typical closed comedones.

Systemic therapy for acne includes:

- antibiotics—tetracycline or erythromycin;
- hormonal therapy—Dianette
- in severe or persistent cases, isotretinoin (Roaccutane, UK; Accutane, USA).

Mild acne

Commonly prescribed preparations for mild acne are those containing 5–10 per cent benzoyl peroxide in a clear gel base (for example Panoxyl 5 and 10, Quinoderm, Benoxyl). These preparations are clear and odourless, and therefore acceptable by both sexes. There may well be some initial mild inflammation and desquamation, particularly in fair-skinned patients. They should be warned of this and encouraged to persevere. True sensitization to benzoyl peroxide is rare, but has been recorded. Topical tetracycline (for example Topicycline, USA and UK) and topical erythromycin (for example Eryderm, USA; Stiemycin, UK) are both cosmetically acceptable and effective.

Topical vitamin A-containing preparations (for example Retin-A gel) are particularly useful if the main problem is closed comedones (whiteheads). Here again some inflammation and irritation is very common.

Topical preparations containing azaleic acid (Skinoren) may help some cases of relatively mild acne.

Moderate acne

Patients with extensive involvement of the facial skin with acne, or those who have not responded to topical therapy, should have a 4–6 month trial of a systemic antibiotic taken in adequate doses. The two antibiotics of choice are tetracycline and erythromycin. Tetracycline or erythromycin should be given in full doses of 1 g/day for at least 3 months. Much the commonest reason for apparent non-response of acne to systemic antibiotic therapy is the prescription of too low a dose for too short a period of time. Tetracycline should be given 30 minutes before meals on an empty stomach and should be washed down with water, not milk which interferes with absorption. Tetracycline should not be given concomitantly with oral iron which will also hinder absorption. Although more expensive than tetracycline doxycycline (Vibramycin, UK) 50 or 100 mg daily is worth considering. It may be used successfully even when conventional tetracycline has failed, possibly due to their absorption and a simpler dosage schedule.

The mode of action of systemic antibiotics in acne is not understood. While a part of their action may be in reducing the *P. acnes* colonization of pilosebaceous follicles, it is also postulated that they may affect chemotaxis of polymorphonuclear leucocytes and thus reduce the inflammatory response.

Side-effects of long-term antibiotic therapy for acne are rare, possibly due to the fact that the patients are otherwise healthy. Overgrowth with *Candida* is unusual. Girls should be warned that tetracycline will be deposited in bones and teeth of a fetus, should they become pregnant, and erythromycin should be given rather than other antibiotics to women who require acne therapy during pregnancy.

For women whose acne persists into their late twenties and thirties, despite adequate topical therapy and repeated courses of systemic antibiotics, a trial of hormonal therapy is justified. Cyproterone acetate is currently available in a dose of 2 mg combined with ethinyl oestradiol as an essential contraceptive (Dianette). If there is no response to a 6 month course of Dianette, these patients should also be considered for retinoid therapy.

Severe or recalcitrant acne

This type of acne can now be well controlled in almost all cases by the use of isotretinoin, a synthetic retinoid which is given systemically. In the UK, this drug is available only on hospital prescription, but in the USA it is freely available. Isotretinoin (Roaccutane, UK; Accutane, USA) appears to have a very specific effect on the pilosebaceous gland and measurements of sebum excretion show a dramatic reduction in outflow of sebum. If the acne-bearing skin is biopsied, the pilosebaceous follicles will be seen to have shrunk to the vestigial structure seen prior to puberty. Isotretinoin is usually prescribed in a dose of 1.0 mg/kg body-weight daily for 4 months, but some patients, usually males with severe back lesions, may need a longer course.

Minor side-effects include dry skin, cheilitis, and, in some cases, a temporary elevation of serum lipids which revert to normal at the end of the course. A few patients on therapy for varying periods of time have been found to have bony abnormalities in the form of hyperostoses and the development of bony spurs around the wrists and ankle areas. By far the most serious problem, however, in the use of isotretinoin is its teratogenicity. It is essential if it is to be prescribed that females understand that pregnancy is absolutely contraindicated. There are reports of fetal abnormalities in children born to women who only took the drug for 1 or 2 weeks. A pregnancy test should be done prior to starting therapy and the patient started on the oral contraceptive 1 month before she starts oral retinoid therapy. This should be continued for 1 month after stopping retinoid therapy. Most patients only need one 4 month course of treatment, but if necessary this can be extended or repeated after 12 months or so.

Table 10.1 outlines the currently available acne treatments.

Acne scarring

The aim of modern acne therapy is to prevent scarring but in some patients scarring has developed before the patient seeks medical advice. In such cases, once all acne activity has ceased, it may be possible to reduce scarring by chemical peeling techniques or dermabrasion, but good results cannot be guaranteed.

Rosacea

Epidemiology and aetiology

Rosacea is relatively common and affects 1 per cent of dermatological outpatients in the UK. It is commoner in women, although men tend to have more severe facial lesions and a higher incidence of the associated complications of keratitis and rhinophyma.

Key Points

The aim of acne treatment is to prevent scarring.

Key Points

Occasionally acne may persist in women into the second and third decades.

Key Points

Complications of rosacea are rhinophyma and keratitis.

Table 10.1.

Management strategies for varying types of acne

Type	Management
Mild teenage acne	Topical benzoyl peroxide or tretinoin
	Advice about non-greasy cosmetics
	Add systemic tetracycline or erythromycin if
	persistent after 3 months topical therapy
Moderately severe acne	Topical benzoyl peroxide
	Tetracycline or erythromycin 1 g/day for a
	minimum of 3 months
	If no response to full doses of antibiotics for
	3–6 months, refer for consideration for
	isotretinoin
Persistent acne in mature	Consider for hormonal therapy
females	(Dianette)
Severe acne	Oral retinoids with oral contraception in
	females

The aetiology of rosacea is unknown. There appears to be an overabundant and hyper-responsive blood supply to the pilosebaceous follicle. Large numbers of the mite *Demodex folliculorum* can be found in the pilosebaceous follicles, but their role in the pathogenesis of rosacea is unknown.

Pathology

Dilatation of the vessels in the papillary dermis and sebaceous hyperplasia are hallmarks. A granulomatous dermal inflammatory infiltrate containing giant cells may be seen in chronic cases.

Clinical features

Most patients first develop rosacea in the third and fourth decades. Flushing and erythema begin typically on the forehead, the bridge of the nose, and cheeks—the so-called butterfly area of the face (Fig.10.7). It may, however, be more widespread and spread to the neck, and occasionally beyond the face and neck areas. Over a period of months or years transient flushing is replaced by persistent erythema on which papules and pustules develop. Unlike acne, there are neither comedones nor seborrhoea.

In severe chronic cases, particularly in males, the sebaceous gland hypertrophy is concentrated on the nose, and produces gross soft tissue overgrowth and

Fig. 10.7 Extensive rosacea.

hypertrophy. The resulting appearance, termed **rhinophyma**, can be disfiguring and at times grotesque (Fig. 10.8).

Ocular involvement is a potentially serious complication. It presents as a sense of 'grittiness' or other discomfort in the eyes. Clinically, there may be a mild blepharitis and conjunctivitis. If keratitis develops, corneal ulceration, vascularization, and visual impairment may also become problems. Rosacea keratitis may develop in those with relatively mild cutaneous lesions.

Perioral dermatitis

It is likely that the condition perioral dermatitis is a variant of rosacea, mainly affecting the chin and cheek area around the mouth. It was relatively common in the 1970s when strong steroids were used inappropriately on the face. Over the past 20 years it has become much less common.

Differential diagnosis

The commoner facial dermatoses to be considered in the differential diagnosis of rosacea include acne vulgaris, light sensitivity, contact dermatitis, lupus erythematosus, and perioral dermatitis. Acne usually affects younger patients and is distinguished by comedones. Both facial photosensitivity and contact dermatitis are more rapid in onset than rosacea and lack pustules. Chronic discoid lupus erythematosus is characterized by discrete scaly lesions, and in the systemic variety of lupus erythematosus the rash has a rapid onset and the patient is generally unwell.

Treatment

Long-term systemic antibiotics, commonly tetracycline, should be prescribed. Oxytetracycline 250 mg four times per day for 2 months reducing to twice daily 30–60 minutes before food for 3–6 months is usually effective (Figs 10.9 and 10.10). Topical metronidazole (Metrogel) is also useful, but rarely effective alone.

Fig. 10.8 Classic rhinophyma complicating rosacea in an elderly male.

Figs 10.9 and 10.10 Patient with rosacea before and after 4 months treatment with systemic tetracycline.

Topical steroids are positively contraindicated.

Severe rhinophyma should be treated surgically. Shaving or excision of the excess soft tissue on the nose and skin grafting can be most effective. This should be done while the patient is receiving systemic tetracycline to reduce the chance of recurrence.

Any patient with rosacea and ocular symptoms, however mild, should be referred to an ophthalmologist without delay. As there is no clear relationship between the severity of cutaneous lesions and the risk of developing ocular lesions, all patients without exception should be asked about ocular symptoms.

Excessive loss of hair

The normal structure and growth cycle of hair are detailed on p. 23–24. When dealing with alopecia, it is useful to remember that normally 80 per cent of scalp hairs are in the anagen phase and 20 per cent in catagen or telogen, and that new follicles cannot be formed in the adult, so that a scarred scalp with irreversible damage to hair follicles will have permanent alopecia.

Hair loss on the scalp may be diffuse or patchy, and the commoner causes are listed in Tables 10.2 and 10.3. Patients rarely complain of hair loss from other sites although it does occur, both in isolation and in association with scalp disorders.

Alopecia areata

Definition

A condition characterized by either generalized or localized sudden hair loss from the scalp or other body sites.

Table 10.2.
Common causes of diffuse hair loss

Male pattern baldness (androgen-dependent baldness)

Telogen effluvium (post-partum, fever, 'stress')

Syphilis

Systemic lupus erythematosus

Endocrine causes: hypothyroidism, hypopituitarism

Nutritional (iron deficiency)

Drug-induced (cytotoxics, anticoagulants, vitamin A, and analogues)

Hair shaft defects (pili torti and monilethrix)

Trichotillomania

Alopecia areata (may be diffuse or localized)

Table 10.3.
Common causes of localized patch hair loss

Alopecia areata

Naevoid abnormalities

Fungal infections, including kerion

Chronic discoid lupus erythematosus

Follicular lichen planus

Traction ('ponytail' hair styles, the use of harsh setting implements)

In some patients there appears to be an underlying genetic predisposition. Certain subgroups are recognized, including one associated with atopy and one with 'autoimmune' disorders (for example thyroid disorders, vitiligo, diabetes). The condition is commoner in children with Downs syndrome.

Alopecia areata is common and accounts for approximately 2 per cent of new cases seen as dermatological out-patients. Most cases are in children or young adults, and the commonest initial sign is one or more well-demarcated, completely bald areas. The affected scalp is normal with no sign of inflammation, scaling, or scarring, but hairs plucked from the margin of the area are often 'club hairs', that is in telogen, and broken hairs in this area resembling exclamation marks (!) are diagnostic (Fig. 10.11).

Complete loss of scalp hair is referred to as **alopecia totalis**, and when all body hair also is lost, the term **alopecia universalis** is applied.

It is not unusual in alopecia areata for the nails to be pitted and ridged.

Fig. 10.11 Alopecia areata. Regular circular lesions appear rapidly. The underlying scalp appears smooth and healthy.

Spontaneous regrowth takes place after an interval of 2–6 months in the majority of cases, but repeated episodes of hair loss are by no means uncommon. Features suggesting that the prognosis must be guarded include associated atopy, loss of eyebrows and lashes, nail change, and multiple lesions at the scalp margins—the so-called ophiasic type.

Diagnosis and treatment

The diagnosis is usually evident on clinical examination but atypical or scaly lesions require mycological examination of scrapings and hair samples to exclude a fungal infection. The use of Wood's light (p. 34) will exclude fungal infection due to most *Microsporum* species and to *Trichophyton schoenleinii*, but not to other species of fungi.

Scalp biopsy is rarely necessary, although the histology is characteristic. There is no loss of hair follicles, but the bulbs lie high in the dermis, are surrounded by lymphoid cells, and produce imperfectly keratinized hair.

As most cases of alopecia areata are self-limiting, the best plan is to reassure the patient and to encourage patience. Sometimes topical steroids or a course of ultraviolet light (UVB), is helpful. Corticosteroids (for example triamcinolone) intralesionally may stimulate the regrowth of a tuft of hair adjacent to the needle track, but the cosmetic result is no improvement on the pre-existing alopecia. In severe and extensive cases prescription of a wig is indicated.

At present the prospects for hair regrowth in persistent alopecia areata are poor. Do not build up false hopes in your patient prior to hospital referral.

Male pattern baldness (androgenic alopecia)

Androgen-dependent loss of scalp hair is extremely common in men and increases with age. There is a genetic component determining the age of onset and severity of the process. A small proportion of post-menopausal women are similarly affected. The main area of loss in men is the crown, with some frontal recession, whereas in women there is fronto-vertical thinning but retention of the frontal hair margin.

In otherwise healthy young men, one can only reassure that there is no underlying disease. The antihypertensive drug minoxidil has been used topically, usually as a 2 per cent solution, in various types of alopecia. In male pattern baldness it does appear in some patients to retard hair loss, but only as long as the topical application continues. In the UK, it is available only on private prescription, and individuals who wish to use it should be informed that it will reduce the rate of hair loss, but that it is not a cure.

When women are concerned by androgenic alopecia, a wig may well be justified once endocrine, drug-induced, and iron deficiency alopecia have been excluded (see below). In the UK, however, there are clear-cut regulations governing the prescription on the National Health Service of either human or synthetic hair wigs. Artificial hair wigs are relatively inexpensive and, unlike those made of human hair, they can be easily washed at home.

Telogen effluvium

Under certain conditions, notably during pregnancy when blood oestrogen is raised, the percentage of hair follicles in anagen rises. As a result, there is a luxuriant head of hair, but after delivery, the follicles held in anagen all enter telogen, and these hairs are therefore shed. This can give rise to significant hair thinning, commonly seen 4–9 months after delivery, but the situation is self-limiting. The diffuse loss of hair which follows high fever, severe illness, or 'stress' results from a similar disturbance of the hair cycle. No specific treatment is available, and after 3–4 months hair follicles resume their normal synchronization.

Miscellaneous causes of hair loss

Syphilis

Some patients with secondary syphilis present with a diffuse 'moth-eaten' pattern of hair loss, but its relationship to the other signs and symptoms at this stage is unclear. Serology is positive. Hair regrowth follows adequate antibiotic therapy.

Systemic lupus erythematosus

Patients with active, usually severe, systemic lupus erythematosus and multi-system involvement may have diffuse generalized hair loss. Unlike the patchy alopecia seen in chronic discoid LE, it is temporary and good regrowth will follow successful systemic therapy.

Endocrine alopecia

Hair loss can accompany hypofunction of the thyroid and pituitary glands. In hypothyroidism hair growth is poor, and the hair shaft is coarse and wire-like. In hypopituitarism total loss of scalp, eyebrow, and secondary sexual hair is frequently seen. This type of alopecia does not always recover after adequate endocrine replacement.

Nutritional alopecia

Chronic iron deficiency anaemia is associated with thin fragile scalp hair (Fig. 10.12). Severe, generalized malnutrition also causes hair loss and premature greying of remaining hair.

Drug-induced alopecia

A large number of cytotoxic drugs cause alopecia and those responsible are listed in Table 10.4. Patients tolerate this form of iatrogenic alopecia much more readily if they are warned beforehand of its inevitability. A well-made wig will greatly improve morale. Heparin and warfarin occasionally cause hair loss, and large doses of vitamin A and the newer synthetic retinoids cause generalized diffuse alopecia.

Fig. 10.12 Hair loss coincident with hypochromic anaemia. Good regrowth was achieved after correction of iron deficiency.

Table 10.4.
Drugs which commonly cause alopecia

Cytotoxic drugs	Cyclophosphamide
	Mercaptopurine derivatives
	Colchicine
	Adriamycin
	Vinca alkaloids
Anticoagulants	Heparin
	Coumarins
Antithyroid drugs	Thiouracil
	Carbimazole
Antituberculous drug	Ethionamide

Topical applications have, as far as is known, only a placebo effect in the above disorders. All patients presenting with generalized hair loss should be investigated for a remediable cause. In a small proportion, usually female, no obvious cause is found and the condition fits no recognized pattern. In these cases, the label 'idiopathic diffuse hair loss' is applied.

Hair shaft defects

A variety of congenital abnormalities of the hair shaft causing undue fragility have been described. Patients present with short broken hair and patchy alopecia. The most common are **monilethrix** (beaded hair) and **pili torti** (twisted

Fig. 10.13 Pili torti. Note the 'spangled' appearance and dry, brittle hair.

hair) (Fig. 10.13). Both of these, and also rarer abnormalities, can be diagnosed on light microscopy of the hair. No topical treatment is available, but gentle handling and a short hair style can be of some value.

Trichotillomania

A compulsive desire to pull, twist, and tug at scalp hair. Extreme forms may be seen in the mentally subnormal and bizarre patterns of hair loss, often unilateral, with clearly visible broken hairs, will suggest the diagnosis.

Naevoid abnormalities

Infants and very young children are occasionally seen with a well-demarcated patch of complete alopecia, and with neither scaling nor fragility of the surrounding hair. This may be due to naevoid abnormalities such as **aplasia cutis**, but histological confirmation of this diagnosis is needed.

Fungal scalp infections

The patient is usually a child with patchy, scaly alopecia and siblings may also be affected. All suspected cases and contacts should be examined under Wood's light (long UV wavelength 365 nm). However, only lesions due to *Microsporum canis* or *M. audouini* will show bright, blue-green fluorescence. Other fungi which commonly cause tinea capitis, such as *Trichophyton verrucosum* and *T. tonsurans*, will not fluoresce in this manner. Scalp scrapings and hairs should be examined microscopically and cultured to demonstrate the fungus.

Sometimes the fungus stimulates an intense inflammatory reaction which forms a large boggy lesion with hair loss and a purulent discharge from the follicles. This constitutes a **kerion** and is usually due to *T. verrucosum* or *T. mentagrophytes* (animal ringworm) (p. 131).

Proven scalp ringworm is treated with full doses of oral griseofulvin or lamisil (p. 131). Hair regrows normally except when lesions such as a kerion leave scarring.

Chronic discoid lupus erythematosus

Patients with facial lesions of CDLE may have similar lesions on the scalp. The alopecia resulting from these lesions is patchy and scaly, and has follicles plugged by scales and an erythematous advancing margin. As it is a scarring process, permanent alopecia will result. Treatment of early lesions and attempts to prevent new lesions developing are discussed on p. 149.

Lichen planus

Occasionally, lichen planus affects the scalp and causes permanent, scarring alopecia (p. 62).

Traction alopecia

Localized hair loss and broken hairs, particularly round the hair margin, may be caused mechanically by tight hair styles (for example 'ponytails') or the use of harsh hair-setting equipment.

Excessive growth of hair

Two terms are applied to excessive hair growth. Hirsutes refers to excess growth of androgen-dependent hair in a male pattern, whereas hypertrichosis is an excess growth of hair in a non-androgenic pattern. Hypertrichosis is seen in both sexes, but hirsutes is restricted to females for, although men are quick to seek help for baldness, they do not complain of excessive growth of hair in a normal distribution.

Hirsutism

Fine vellus hair covers much of the body in both sexes and can be induced by androgens to transform into coarse terminal hair. The causes of hirsutism can be grouped under general headings as in Table 10.5.

Key Points

Hirsutism may be due to an endocrine disfunction resulting in an elevated androgen level or (more commonly) it may be idiopathic.

Table 10.5.
Causes of hirsutism

Adrenal: Cushing's syndrome, virilizing tumours, congenital adrenal hyperplasia
Pituitary: acromegaly
Ovarian: polycystic ovaries, virilizing tumours, gonadal dysgenesis
Turner's syndrome
Iatrogenic: due to androgenic drugs
Idiopathic: target or end-organ hypersensitivity—much the commonest cause

Women with hirsutism complain of hair growth in the beard area (Fig. 10.14), around the nipples, and in a male pattern on the abdomen. They are more likely to be dark-haired and the problem appears to be commoner in certain racial groups, for example those of Mediterranean origin. Hirsutism can cause remarkable distress to a healthy woman and psychological disturbance with depression is common in younger women, even those in whom the condition is relatively mild.

Investigation and treatment

The aim in investigating the hirsute patient is to exclude an underlying, remediable endocrine cause. Although many tests of adrenal, ovarian, and

Fig. 10.14 Hirsuties. Excessive growth of facial hair on the chin of a female.

pituitary function are available, the young woman who is menstruating regularly and has had one or more successful pregnancies, probably requires little in the way of endocrine assessment and is likely to fall into the idiopathic group, in which to date only marginally elevated levels of plasma testosterone have been found. It would appear that the fault in this group, by far the largest, lies in the hypersensitivity of the hair follicle as an end-organ of androgen stimulation.

Full endocrine assessment is, however, essential in patients with amenorrhoea, scanty, irregular periods, or other signs of excess androgen stimulation. This assessment should include estimation of plasma cortisol, free testosterone, of sex hormone binding globulin, FSH, LH, and ultrasound of ovaries and adrenals.

Therapy for those with no demonstrable remediable cause consists of physical methods of hair removal. Shaving, bleaching, and depilatory creams are all used, but the most satisfactory method is waxing as it also removes a large part of the hair shaft lying under the skin surface. Most patients find a professional demonstration of the technique helpful. If systemic therapy is necessary, Dianette may be effective, but must be used for 6 months before any response can be anticipated.

Hypertrichosis

Hypertrichosis may be either congenital or acquired.

Congenital varieties are frequently associated with melanocytic naevi, while lumbosacral hypertrichosis ('faun tail') should alert the paediatrician or obstetrician to the possibility of spina bifida occulta.

Acquired hypertrichosis is most commonly drug-induced, although porphyria (p. 266) and endocrine disorders (thyroid dysfunction and anorexia nervosa) are recognized causes. Drugs in current use which can cause hypertrichosis include diazoxide, diphenylhydantoin, penicillamine, and the psoralens. If the offending drug is withdrawn, the excessive hair growth will cease.

Disorders of the nails

The normal anatomy of the nail is described on p. 26. Factors controlling nail growth are poorly understood but the average time taken for a finger-nail to grow out is 6–12 months and for a toe-nail 18–24 months. These figures increase with age and there is seasonal variation, with some acceleration in the summer months. Individual nails also vary in their growth rates, with the thumb nail growing relatively rapidly.

Although nail biopsy through both nail and nail bed is feasible it is more traumatic than a routine skin biopsy, so fewer histological specimens from nail disorders than from other sites have been studied. Diagnosis is, therefore, commonly based on clinical appearances.

Nail involvement is common in many skin diseases: for example, onycholysis and pitting in psoriasis, discoloration and crumbling in fungal infections, pitting and ridging in chronic dermatitis, and a more severe dystrophy in lichen planus. These are all discussed with the relevant diseases.

Nail disorders can, however, occur in isolation and can be either congenital or acquired.

Congenital nail disorders

The nail-patella syndrome

This condition is transmitted by autosomal dominant inheritance. The patellae and some of the nails are rudimentary or absent. The thumb nails are usually involved.

Pachyonychia congenita

Misshapen, hypertrophic nails are present from birth and there may also be associated mucous membrane abnormalities. The condition is inherited by autosomal dominant transmission (Fig. 10.15).

Fig. 10.15 Pachyonychia congenita. Note the gross abnormality of all toenails in both father and son. Finger-nails were similarly affected.

Acquired nail defects

Beau's lines

Transverse ridges on the nails due to temporary interference with nail formation.

These lines are commonly seen during convalescence from a variety of severe disease states, for example pneumonia and other conditions causing prolonged fever. The condition is self-limiting.

Koilonychia

Loss of the normal nail contour resulting in a flat or even depressed surface.

Nails of this shape are commonly slow-growing and brittle. They are most commonly associated with hypochromic anaemia and correction of iron deficiency may be followed by return to normal growth of the nails.

Finger clubbing

An exaggeration of the normal nail curve associated with loss of the normal angle between nail and posterior nail fold.

In adults this appearance is commonly seen in those with pulmonary pathology. If of slow onset, chronic respiratory infection and bronchiectasis is a likely cause, and, if of more rapid onset, the possibility of carcinoma of the lung must be considered. In young people clubbing and nail changes may be seen in association with cyanotic congenital heart disease.

The mechanisms giving rise to these conformational changes of the finger tips are not understood. The resultant lesions may be both disfiguring and painful.

Paronychia

Acute paronychia is commonly due to staphylococcal infection and consists of an acutely inflamed posterior nail fold with a purulent discharge. There is frequently a history of trauma. Response to an appropriate systemic antibiotic is prompt.

Chronic paronychia is more persistent and troublesome. Usually, several nails are affected and show striking loss of the cuticle with tender, bolstered, posterior nail folds. If bacterial in origin, the likely organisms are *Pseudomonas pyocanea* and *Proteus vulgaris*, but frequently the cause is *Candida*, usually *C. albicans*. Persistent immersion of the hands in water is a common predisposing factor, so that housewives and barmaids are particularly at risk.

Treatment should be directed at organisms identified on culture. *Candida albicans* usually responds well to nystatin suspension or amphotericin B lotion. A useful paint is freshly prepared sulphacetamide 15 per cent in 50 per cent ethanol applied four times daily. Griseofulvin is not of value in these cases.

If the paronychia is shown to be due to *Candida,* and does not respond to topical therapy, a 2–4-week course of ketoconazole (Nizoral) 200 mg/day is justified. The drug must not be given to pregnant women and liver function must be monitored.

If wet work must be done, cotton gloves under rubber gloves must be worn and changed frequently.

Herpetic whitlow

Acute paronychia due to herpes simplex is an occupational hazard in doctors and nurses. It is discussed and illustrated on p. 123.

Paronychial tumours

Warts are frequently found around the nails and may be extremely painful due to pressure on the nail bed. They respond slowly to conventional therapy (p. 116).

Malignant tumours may also occur in this site, the most serious being a malignant melanoma. Any patient with a bleeding or pigmented nodule in the region of a nail should be referred without delay for a diagnostic biopsy and definitive treatment (p. 294).

Iatrogenic nail abnormalities

Systemic drug therapy can cause a variety of nail changes. Tetracycline-induced photosensitivity can lead to nail loss and long-term ingestion of tetracyclines may cause yellow nails. Antimalarial drugs cause blue and blue-black discoloration of the nail beds.

Disorders of the sweat glands

The sweat glands are of two sorts. The **eccrine glands** are concerned with thermoregulation and are distributed over the entire body surface. The **apocrine glands**, found chiefly in the axillae and groins, have no apparent function in man, but appear to be stimulated by emotional stress and contribute to axillary odour.

Eccrine gland disorders

Miliaria (prickly heat)

In the UK miliaria is a rarity, except in a heat wave or the tropical environment of a neonatal nursery. In subtropical or tropical climates it is common, especially in recent arrivals who have not yet acclimatized. Sweat duct obstruction due to high humidity is the cause.

Clinically, there is an acute papulo-vesicular eruption, usually on the trunk. It is itchy, and scratching often leads to crusting and secondary infection.

Treatment is palliative, unless the humidity can be adequately reduced. This is feasible, desirable, and effective in the nursery, but less so in the tropics if no air conditioning is available. A shake lotion, such as calamine lotion BP, can be soothing.

Hyperhidrosis

Over-production of eccrine sweat can be due to heat or to emotional stimuli, but is rarely due to endocrinological or neurological disorders. The nature of the stimulus determines whether the hyperhidrosis is localized or generalized. When localized, the palms, soles, and axillae are the usual sites. Malodour of the feet and axillae due to bacterial overgrowth is common and distressing. Hyperhidrosis of the palms can incapacitate those whose work involves writing and handling of paper.

In generalized hyperhidrosis it is important first to exclude underlying systemic disease. Propranolol 20–40 mg four times per day may be useful.

For localized hyperhidrosis, topical preparations are generally more effective, but may require supplementation with systemic therapy. A paint consisting of 20 per cent aluminium chloride hexahydrate made up in 70 per cent alcohol applied overnight to clean, dry palms, soles, and axillae is effective, mainly in the axillae. If the axillae only are affected, surgical excision of ellipses of skin 2–4 inches long from the vault of the axilla can be dramatically effective. The areas of maximum sweat production should be removed and they can be identified prior to surgery by starch-iodine application. This entire procedure can be done as an out-patient under local anaesthesia.

Chemical or surgical sympathectomy are also helpful in some cases, and a trial of chemical sympathectomy is recommended.

Apocrine gland disorder

Hidradenitis suppurativa

Deep-seated inflammatory lesions chiefly in the axillae and groins (Fig. 10.16).

A functional and structural abnormality of apocrine sweat glands is the cause. Patients do not have normal communication between the secretory and excretory

Fig. 10.16 Hidradenitis suppurativa. Recurrent infection in the apocrine glands causes development of fibrotic scar tissue.

components of the gland. They present with multiple, deeply-situated pustules and abscesses which, in time, damage the dermis and lead to deep scarring. Deep, cord-like fibrotic lesions may restrict movement.

Long-term systemic antibiotic therapy given for a minimum of 3–6 months may give temporary relief. In some patients hidradenitis suppurativa is associated with severe acne. In patients with this combination the use of oral isotretinoin (Roaccutane) given orally in a dose of 1 mg/kg/day for 3 months may be of therapeutic value. In women of child-bearing age adequate contraception is essential.

Surgical excision of the affected area with skin grafting, if required, is the most useful method of permanently eradicating this difficult problem.

Discussion of problem cases

Case 10.1

This young woman is older than the normal age for presentation with acne vulgaris, although late onset acne is becoming commoner especially in females. Cosmetic allergies do not usually present with papules. Erythema and itch would be more common presenting features of a cosmetic allergy.

The description suggests rosacea, and on questioning the patient she agrees that she flushes easily when in a warm room and after eating spicy foods. Careful examination establishes that she has papules and one or two pustules but no comedones (blackheads) are present.

This patient, therefore, requires treatment with a systemic antibiotic, probably tetracycline, for 3–6 months. If there is any possibility of her wishing to start a family, an alternative antibiotic should be used because of the fact that tetracycline will stain the developing teeth of the foetus. She should also be given topical metronidazole gel, and she should be specifically asked not to use any topical steroids on her face.

On this regime this patient's papules cleared although she continues to flush easily in a warm environment.

Case 10.2

Conditions to be considered in the differential diagnosis of hair loss in children are fungal infections, alopecia areata, and trichotillomania. Tinea capitis (p. 131) must be excluded particularly if the child has had contact with animals and if there is any scaling or itch on the scalp. Neither of these were present in this boy's case, but taking some clippings and scrapings for mycological assessment is good practice in this type of presentation. The pattern of hair loss, with several circular patches involved, does not suggest trichotillomania where the usual presentation is of one area of hair loss with broken hairs around the area of visiible alopecia. The pattern strongly suggests alopecia areata.

Treatment of alopecia areata is difficult. Both the boy and his mother should be told that the hair will re-grow in time, but that it is impossible to predict when this will occur. This may be accelerated by use of a moderately potent topical steroid or by a course of ultraviolet radiation.

The prognosis for re-growth following a first attack of alopecia areata is good, but after the second or subsequent episodes, it is wise to be rather more cautious about the likelihood of complete re-growth. Patients who have atopy in addition to alopecia areata have a poorer prognosis for re-growth.

This boy had no history of atopy and his hair re-grew well over a period of 6 months.

Case 10.3

Persistent, recurrent infection is one of the presenting features of several of the immunodeficiency syndromes, but these infections usually start in early childhood, not after puberty as has been the case with this young man. This patient is otherwise fit, and has no lesions on any other body site. This anatomic distribution suggests an apocrine gland abnormality, and the age at onset and clinical description suggest hidradenitis suppurativa. The patient should have full doses of an appropriate systemic antibiotic, determined on bacteriological sensitivity tests, for at least 3–4 months or until complete clearance of the lesions. If this is not effective, then he should be considered for surgical excision of the areas with skin grafting if necessary.

Nine months later, after a further unsuccessful trial of systemic antibiotics, this young man had the worst affected axilla surgically treated with an excellent result. He himself requested surgery for the second axilla, and is currently relatively free of problems.

Projects

1. Consider the risk–benefit ratio of isotretinoin for the management of acne. Review the literature on the reported teratogenicity, and consider how you would describe this drugs benefits and problems to a group of 17 year old students with severe acne?

2. Review the causes of hair loss associated with systemic disease, and useful investigations. Which investigations are likely to be the most cost effective?

Further reading

Cunliffe, W.J. (1989). *Acne*. Martin Dunitz, London.

Berker, D., Baran, R., and Dawber, R.P.R. (1995). *Diseases of the nails and their management*. Blackwell Scientific Publications, Oxford.

Rooke, A.J. and Dawber, R.P.R. (1983). Disorders of the hair and scalp. Blackwell Scientific Publications, Oxford.

A comprehensive account of abnormalities of the hair follicle.

Blistering diseases

- Pemphigus
- Bullous pemphigoid
- Dermatitis herpetiformis
- Epidermolysis bullosa
- Erythema multiforme
- Stevens—Johnson syndrome
- Staphylococcal scalded skin syndrome
- Papular urticaria
- Urticaria pigmentosa

Problem cases

Case 11.1

You are doing a six month obstetrics post prior to entering general practice. On a Saturday night a young, unmarried woman is admitted to the labour ward and delivers a female child who is otherwise healthy but who has small blisters on both feet and one hand. What conditions must be considered in the differential diagnosis of blistering in a neonate, and what investigations should be carried out? What is the likely diagnosis in this situation?

Case 11.2

You are asked to visit a retirement home because an 86-year-old female has an itchy eruption on her limbs which has not settled with topical 1 per cent hydrocortisone cream. Because of the pressure of other commitments, you do not manage to visit the home until 48 hours later, by which time the patient has developed blisters on inflamed skin of her upper arms and thighs. She is on multiple drugs including antihypertensives, non-steroid anti-inflammatories, regular laxatives, and hypnotics. What is the likely diagnosis and how would you confirm it?

Introduction

Skin diseases in which blisters are a predominant or presenting feature are relatively rare but important, because in both children and adults they may be the first sign of a severe and potentially fatal problem. In adults the main group of blistering problems is associated with autoantibody formation, while in children, the rare but important group of genodermatoses, epidermolysis bullosa is associated mainly with mechanical defects in and around the basement membrane zone.

Blisters may arise either because of disruption of the desmosomes between keratinocytes in the epidermis, causing an intraepidermal blister, or because of a defect in the basement membrane zone between the epidermis and dermis, leading to a subepidermal blister.

Accurate diagnosis of blistering problems requires a biopsy of a small, newly formed lesion and also a piece of perilesional skin frozen for immunopathological studies. In some situations, electron microscopy will also be needed.

Pemphigus

Definition

A group of disorders characterized by the development of autoantibodies against desmocollins and desmogleins in the epidermis, giving rise to superficial erosions

Key Points

> Blistering diseases are rare but important as they may be a sign of a severe, and potentially fatal, problem.

Key Points

> Think of pemphigus in severe persistent oral ulcers not due to candida or herpes.

and blisters on both epidermal and mucosal surfaces. Desmocollins and desmogleins are transmembrane desmosomal glycoproteins and are members of the cadherin gene superfamily.

There are four varieties of pemphigus:

- pemphigus vulgaris
- pemphigus vegetans
- pemphigus foliaceus
- pemphigus erythematosus.

Pemphigus vulgaris is the commonest variety of pemphigus, and usually begins with shallow erosions and easily ruptured blisters on mucosal surfaces.

Pemphigus vegetans has striking papillomatous proliferations in the flexures (Fig. 11.1).

Pemphigus foliaceus in Europe and North America is a mild, superficial variant (Fig. 11.2). It is endemic in parts of South America, and there is evidence that it may be caused by an infective agent. This form of pemphigus does not affect children.

Pemphigus erythematosus shares some of the features of pemphigus and of lupus erythematosus. Blisters tend to form on sun-exposed sites, and the patient has both pemphigus and antinuclear antibodies.

Pathology and immunopathology

The main pathological feature of all types of pemphigus is the presence of a superficial, fluid-filled blister within the epidermis.

In pemphigus vulgaris the base of this blister is formed by the basal cells of the epidermis which remain attached to the basement membrane zone; in the

Fig. 11.1 Pemphigus vegetans. Note warty lesions with minimal blister on lower legs.

Fig. 11.2 Pemphigus foliaceus. Note very superficial blistering with scaling on light exposed site.

other varieties the blister may be even more superficial, forming just under the stratum corneum. Individual keratinocytes detach from their neighbours and float free in the blister, a process called **acantholysis**.

Immunopathology shows the presence of autoantibodies directed against the epidermal intercellular material. These autoantibodies are both tissue-fixed—on the patient's perilesional skin—and circulating in the patient's serum. This antibody is tissue-specific but not species-specific, and thus the substrate used for detecting autoantibodies in the patient's serum need not be human tissue, but any source of stratified squamous epithelium such as guinea-pig lip or primate oesophagus. The autoantibody is usually an IgG, and complement is also fixed at the site (Fig. 11.3).

Fig. 11.3 Indirect immunofluorescence test in pemphigus vulgaris. The patient's serum has been layered on mucous membrane substrate and subsequently treated with fluorescein-conjugated antihuman IgG. Specific staining of the intercellular substance is observed.

Circulating pemphigus antibody titres correlate with disease activity, and high-titre serum can induce pemphigus-like lesions both in experimental animals and in organ culture. These observations are supporting evidence that pemphigus is an autoimmune disease, and that the autoantibody causes the disease, and is not just a secondary development.

Clinical features

Pemphigus vulgaris frequently begins insidiously with the slow development of raw areas and shallow erosions on the mucous membranes (Fig. 11.4). Involvement of the skin tends to come later (Fig. 11.5). The patient may, therefore, complain first of mouth ulcers or genital discomfort. The lesions do not itch, but can be very painful. Blisters may develop on both mucous membrane

Fig. 11.4 Oral lesions in a case of early pemphigus vulgaris.

Fig. 11.5 Lesions on the back of a patient with pemphigus vulgaris. Shallow erosions are seen, and healing lesions show some increase in pigmentation.

and skin, but they are quickly denuded by friction or pressure, leaving a raw surface. This feature reflects the thin blister roof of the intraepidermal blister in pemphigus, in contrast to the greater resilience of the subepidermal blister in bullous pemphigoid and dermatitis herpetiformis. Clinically normal skin may display the **Nikolsky sign**—if lateral pressure is put on the skin surface with the thumb the epidermis appears to slide over the underlying dermis.

Secondary infection and disturbance of fluid and electrolyte balance are common complications of untreated pemphigus which, prior to the introduction of corticosteroid therapy, was regularly fatal.

Diagnosis and treatment

The diagnosis should be confirmed and treatment started without delay. Table 11.1 lists conditions which may cause diagnostic confusion. Systemic steroids will be needed. The exact dose depends on the patient's size and disease severity, but the range is 60–100 mg of prednisolone or equivalent per day. Once control has been achieved and no fresh blisters are developing, the dose can be slowly reduced by 20–30 mg/week. A maintenance dose is usually necessary, possibly for life, to prevent recurrence. This should be kept as low as possible, preferably using an alternate-day regime to minimize steroid side-effects. In some patients the addition of an immunosuppressive agent, such as azathioprine or cyclophosphamide, will allow further reduction of the steroid dose. Oral cyclosporin may also be useful. Plasmapheresis is occasionally needed in severe cases.

Topical therapy is mainly symptomatic, and aimed at protecting the raw areas and decreasing the incidence of secondary infection. Vaseline-impregnated gauze dressings are kind to the patient and the lesions should be managed in the same way as burns. In severe cases a ripple bed, burns hammock, or net bed may be valuable.

Although the disease is usually controllable, it rarely remits spontaneously. Consequently, the patient will probably have to remain on systemic steroids for life and will therefore require careful surveillance for steroid-induced side-effects.

Consider the possibility of early pemphigus in any patient with persistent, severe oral erosions. Sending a serum sample for autoantibody testing will confirm your suspicion.

Bullous pemphigoid

Definition

A blistering disorder characterized by large, tense blisters on an erythematous base.

Bullous pemphigoid is found mainly in those aged 60 or older. It is therefore becoming a commoner disease in Europe and North America as the average age of the population increases. All those who are involved in caring for the elderly should be aware of the presenting features.

Table 11.1.

The differential diagnosis of blistering diseases in the adult

	Site	History	Histology	Immunology	Other tests
Pemphigus	Mucous membranes, and trunk	Insidious onset	Intraepidermal blister	Direct IgG C_3 Circulating IgG	
Pemphigoid	Upper arms and thighs	Blisters on eczematous base	Subepidermal blister	Fixed Ig and C_3 at dermo-epidermal junction. Circulating IgG	
Dermatitis herpetiformis	Scalp, scapular area, elbows, buttocks	Pruritus + + +	Subepidermal blister	IgA in papillary dermis	Subtotal villous atrophy on jejunal biopsy
Erythema multiforme	Hands and feet	Target lesions blister	Subepidermal	Negative	Occasionally drug or viral history
Mechanical blisters	Site of trauma	Friction, e.g. marching, poorly fitting shoes	Subepidermal blister	Negative	
Atypical herpes simplex or zoster	Variable	Prodromal pain and tingling	Balloon degeneration within the epidermis	Rising specific antibody titre	Electron microscopy to demonstrate virus particles
Herpes zoster	Linear dermatome distribution	Pain and tingling: may be severe	Intraepidermal balloon degeneratioin	Rising specific antibody titre	
Porphyria cutanea tarda	Sun-exposed sites	Sun exposure, minor friction, and trauma	Subepidermal blister	Autofluorescence of porphyrins	Raised uroporphyrin levels

Pathology

The blister is subepidermal, formed between the dermis and epidermis. As the entire thickness of the epidermis forms the roof of the blisters, they are relatively resilient and may remain intact for several days.

As with pemphigus, tissue-fixed and circulating autoantibodies have been demonstrated, suggesting that the disease may have an autoimmune pathogenesis. In bullous pemphigoid, immunoglobulin and complement are deposited in the lamina lucida of the basement membrane in a linear band, and there is a circulating antibody specific to this site (Fig. 11.6).

Fig. 11.6 Indirect immunofluorescence test using bullous pemphigoid serum on primate oesophagus as a substrate. A clear band of IgG is seen in the basement membrane zone.

Fig. 11.7 Blisters of bullous pemphigoid. Large, tense, raised lesions are seen on an erythematous eczematized base.

Clinical features

Patients are usually elderly and present with large, tense blisters, mainly on the upper arms and thighs (Fig. 11.7 and 11.8). These arise on an eczematous base and there is itch rather than pain. Some spontaneous haemorrhage into the blisters is not uncommon. Oral lesions are less frequent than in pemphigus but should be sought.

Treatment

Systemic steroid therapy is usually necessary, but unlike pemphigus, it may be possible to discontinue this after 2 to 3 years. A starting dose of 60–100 mg prednisolone or equivalent should be gradually reduced to the minimum which will control the disease. Further dose reduction may be possible if immunosuppressive agents are added to the regimen. In milder cases it has recently been suggested that oral dapsone in doses of 50–150 mg/day may be effective therapy.

Although bullous pemphigoid does not carry as high an immediate morbidity and mortality as pemphigus, the elderly do not tolerate steroid or cytotoxic therapy well, and there is a high incidence of treatment-induced complications in bullous pemphigoid patients, some of them fatal. These patients therefore need careful supervision.

Dermatitis herpetiformis

Definition

An intensely itchy, blistering condition associated with a gluten-sensitive enteropathy.

Dermatitis herpetiformis (DH) affects a younger age group than the other two blistering disorders. Patients present in the third and fourth decade and males are more commonly affected.

Key Points

Dermatitis herpetiformis can be misdiagnosed as scabies.

Fig. 11.8 Bullous pemphigoid showing typical involvement of upper limb.

Fig. 11.9 Immunopathology of dermatitis herpetiformis. This section of perilesional skin has been treated with FITC-labelled antihuman IgG. Note fluorescence marked with arrow in dermal papilla.

Pathology

The blisters are subepidermal and are small by comparison with the larger lesions in bullous pemphigoid. There are frequently aggregates of leucocytes in so-called 'microabscesses' at tips of the dermal papillae flanking the blister.

No circulating antibody has yet been consistently found in DH patients, but direct immunofluorescence of the skin around lesions will reveal the presence of IgA and sometimes complement in the dermal papillae (Fig. 11.9).

Clinical features

Patients complain of an intense, burning itch on the affected sites, commonly the scalp, scapular area, buttocks, and elbows (Figs 11.10 and 11.11). Very small blisters may be found, but as they are quickly excoriated, raw papules may be the only lesions seen.

Most patients will have no overt signs or symptoms of malabsorption and opinion is divided as to whether or not a jejunal biopsy should be performed in this situation. There is no doubt that a gluten free diet, if rigorously followed, will help most patients whether or not they have gastrointestinal symptoms.

Treatment

Dermatitis herpetiformis does not respond to systemic steroids. Itch will be controlled by dapsone in doses of 50–150 mg/day, but careful haematological monitoring is necessary, as a haemolytic anaemia may develop. Oral Sulphapyridine by mouth is a second-line drug, the dose being 0.5–1.0 g/day. Other, newer sulphonamides are less effective.

Topical steroid-antibiotic combinations (for example vioform-hydrocortisone, β-methasone 17-valerate with chinoform, or aureomycin) are useful supplements to systemic therapy.

Fig. 11.10 Dermatitis herpetiformis. Small grouped blisters are seen.

Fig. 11.11 Dermatitis herpetiformis showing intensely itchy vesicles and blisters on the shoulder area.

As this is a chronic disease, treatment may need to be life-long.

The epidermolysis bullosa group of blistering disorders

This group of blistering disorders comprise the rare but serious group of mechano-bullous disorders. They usually present at birth or in infancy, but cause problems thereafter throughout life. They are genetically determined and range from relatively mild problems to life threatening and life ruining conditions. As prenatal diagnosis is now available for couples known to be at risk, it is essential to be aware of the features of these diseases, so that if a neonate presents with blisters an accurate pathological diagnosis can be made on which future genetic counselling can be based.

The main varieties are:

- **epidermolysis bullosa simplex**—mainly autosomal dominant;
- **junctional epidermolysis bullosa**—autosomal recessive;
- **dystrophic epidermolysis bullosa**—both autosomal dominant, and autosomal recessive varieties.

A tentative diagnosis can be made on the basis of a family history, clinical examination, and light microscopic examination of a skin biopsy, but a definitive diagnosis is essential for genetic counselling and for this electron microscopy is required to locate the site of the damage at ultrastructural level.

Epidermolysis bullosa simplex

Twelve variants of EB simplex are currently recognized, the majority inherited by autosomal dominant transmission. The pathological damage in this variety lies within the epidermis and consists of a split through the cytoplasm of the basal cells. Thus, there is true cell lysis. The molecular defect lies in defective genes coding for keratins 5 and 14 which are found preferentially in the basal layer. Blisters may be present at birth, but often the disease first becomes apparent when the child starts to walk or crawl, and develops mild blistering and desquamation on knees, hands, feet, and other sites of friction (Fig. 11.12). These blisters quickly rupture and heal with no subsequent scarring. Other ectodermal structures (hair, teeth, and nails) are unaffected and mucous membranes, although occasionally involved, do not show gross changes. There is little tendency to remission in later childhood or adult life.

Junctional epidermolysis bullosa (Herlitz type, epidermolysis bullosa letalis)

All seven currently recognized variants of this type are inherited by autosomal recessive transmission and the basic abnormality appears to lie in the

Fig. 11.12 Epidermolysis bullosa simplex. This child develops blisters on sites of friction. Healing is rapid without scarring.

hemidesmosomes. Defective genes normally coding for bullous pemphigoid antigen and laminin have recently been identified in the generalized, atrophic, benign variant of this EB subtype. This results in the development of a split at the level of the lamina lucida. The overlying epidermis appears normal and there is no obvious loss of cohesion between the cells. The base of the blister is formed by an intact basal lamina still firmly adherent to the dermis.

Clinical abnormality may be present at birth either as blisters, often around the nails, or raw denuded areas, with little tendency to heal. Mucous membranes may be severely involved, and the teeth are commonly abnormal. A high proportion of these children die in infancy.

Fig. 11.13 Epidermolysis bullosa of the dominant dystrophic type. Note extensive blistering with scarring on knees and shins.

Dystrophic epidermolysis bullosa

There are at present 11 recognized variants and inheritance can be either autosomal dominant or autosomal recessive (Table 11.2). The abnormality consists of defective anchoring fibrils connecting the basal lamina to the dermis and a subepidermal blister results. Production of collagen type 7 is also reduced or absent, and this contributes to the physical weakness of this area. In the dominant varieties, in later infancy or early childhood bullae form on friction sites and heal with scarring. Milia may be seen in these scars, which tend to become keloidal or hyperplastic (Fig 11.13). Hair and teeth develop normally.

In the recessive types, there is also a defect of anchoring fibrils, Large bullae are present at birth, and they heal with scarring which is associated with the formation of webs between fingers and eventually a useless fist Mucous membranes, hair, nails (Fig. 11.14), and teeth may all be abnormal, and there are reports of the development of squamous carcinoma on the scar sites.

Fig. 11.14 Dystrophic epidermolysis bullosa. Note the loss of finger-nails. This 5-year-old child already has web formation between the digits.

Table 11.2

Current subdivisions of the epidermolysis bullosa group of disorders

Type	Number of varieties	Inheritance	Site of blister	Specific defect	Clinical features
Simplex	12	Mainly autosomal dominant	Basal cells	Keratins 5 and 14	Mainly friction induced blisters on hands and feet
Junctional	7	All autosomal recessive	Lamina lucida	Hemidesmosomes	Extensive blistering of skin. Mucosal involvement
Dystrophic	11	Mixed	Below basement membrane	Anchoring fibrils Type 7 collagen	Varied loss of nails and scarring

Treatment and prenatal diagnosis of epidermolysis bullosa

Children with epidermolysis bullosa should be managed by a team with experience of the problem. Skilled nursing care is vital for the more severe forms, and membership of Debra, the patient support group, is very worthwhile. Once an accurate histological diagnosis has been established by electron microscopy, protective measures should be taken in all cases to prevent friction bullae. Infants who are still crawling should have padded trousers, and special soft footwear will be needed. A trial of systemic steroids is worthwhile in the junctional and dystrophic varieties. Specialist dental care will be needed for children with oral lesions. Occupational therapy may delay the development of contractures or webs in the autosomal recessive dystrophic variety, but the prognosis for both survival and the ability to lead an independent adult life must be guarded in these varieties of the disorder.

It is important that genetic counselling be offered to parents of children with epidermolysis bullosa. This entails making an accurate diagnosis, and constructing a full and accurate family tree going back at least two generations. Parents can then be given a reliable estimate of the risks of producing another affected child, and informed that prenatal diagnosis is possible by fetal skin biopsy.

The technique of fetal skin biopsy to diagnose epidermolysis bullosa in mothers who are at risk is now relatively well established. Chorionic villus biopsy is taken at around 9 weeks gestation and DNA analysis performed. If the test is positive for one of the more severe types of epidermolysis bullosa, the parents can decide whether or not the pregnancy should proceed.

Erythema multiforme

Definition

An erythematous disorder characterized by annular, target lesions which may develop into frank blisters.

Aetiology

Erythema multiforme (EM) is a cutaneous reaction pattern which may be provoked by viral infection, commonly herpes simplex, by bacterial infection, by drug ingestion, and many other stimuli. In many cases, however, no aetiological or precipitating factor can be identified. In the bullous lesions of EM, the blister forms at the dermo–epidermal junction, and there is necrosis and destruction of the overlying epidermis.

Clinical features

The lesions are most commonly seen on the hands and feet and initially present as raised erythematous plaques which expand laterally to give the classic 'iris lesion' or 'target lesion' appearance (Fig. 11.15).

Severe involvement of the eyes and mucosal surfaces is termed the **Stevens–Johnson syndrome.**

Toxic epidermal necrolysis (TEN) (Fig. 11.16) is also a severe variant of EM with extensive shedding of epidermis but less mucosal involvement. Identification and removal of the cause is important, and all suspect drugs should be withdrawn. A few patients will settle on bed rest and topical steroid applications, but the majority will require a short course of systemic steroids over a period of 10–14 days.

Fig. 11.15 Erythema multiforme on the leg, note the presence of target lesions.

Fig. 11.16 Toxic epidermal necrolysis. Note extensive erythema and early development of blisters and raw areas on the legs.

Fig. 11.17 Staphylococcal scalded skin syndrome. Note the shearing of the epidermis, and lack of inflammation of the surrounding skin.

Staphylococcal scalded skin syndrome

Staphylococcal scalded skin syndrome is a blistering disorder caused by an epidermolytic toxin of certain phage types of *Staphylococcus aureus* which cleaves the epidermis at the level of the granular layer. The condition is commoner in children than in adults, and is seen as rapidly expanding, very shallow blisters, which quickly rupture, leaving painful, raw areas (Figs 11.17 and 11.18). All patients should be swabbed for bacteriological sensitivities, and should then be started on a systemic antistaphylococcal antibiotic without delay. This can be changed, if necessary, once bacteriological sensitivities are known.

Papular urticaria (bites)

Although papular urticaria is frequently seen in paediatric skin clinics, a high proportion of affected children are managed either by parents or the family doctor.

Characteristically, the lesions are grouped and occur in crops (Fig. 11.19). Morphologically, they are tender, erythematous papules or small blisters. They are quickly scratched and subsequently become secondarily infected.

In a high proportion of cases fleas or mites are to blame, but tact must be used when persuading parents that this is so.

Suitable treatment of established lesions is a topical antipruritic such as crotamiton or 2 per cent menthol in calamine cream. Prevention of further crops is difficult and depends on eliminating the causative factor. The child's bedding and family pets should be treated with an insecticidal dusting powder.

Urticaria pigmentosa

Definition

An eruption due to focal aggregation of mast cells in the dermis, seen usually in infancy.

Although both children and adults are affected, urticaria pigmentosa is most often seen in infancy. The lesions are multiple erythematous weals which may blister and are provoked by minor trauma or a warm bath. The lesions resolve, leaving some melanin pigmentation (Fig. 11.20). Biopsy will reveal foci of mast cells: these degranulate on trauma, releasing vasoactive substances which elicit the lesion.

Spontaneous improvement throughout infancy and childhood is usual. Treatment consists of avoiding trauma until remission occurs. Antihistamines are not indicated.

In severe cases of urticaria pigmentosa, a trial of oral sodium cromoglycate (Nalcrom) is justified as there are reports of a good response, presumably due to mast cell stabilization.

Discussion of problem cases

Case 11.1

The differential diagnosis of blisters in the newborn range from benign and transient to serious life threatening problems. The minor problems include trauma from the pressure of delivery, particularly if forceps have been applied, and low grade infection, either staphylococcal or viral. More serious concern is that of epidermolysis bullosa group of disorders, some of which are potentially lethal. The majority of these present as blisters at birth.

The blisters in this child's case persisted and extended over the first few days of life, and bacteriological and virological culture showed no growth. A biopsy of a small fresh blister with immunopathology and electron microscopy was therefore arranged. The ultrastructural findings showed that the child had a blister which was forming as a result of a split through the basal cells of the epidermis. This pattern confirms the diagnosis of the most benign type of epidermolysis bullosa, EB simplex. The clinical pattern suggested an autosomal dominant variety of this condition. What genetic counselling can be offered in this situation? What management plan would you devise for this baby? What is the prognosis?

Case 11.2

Pruritus in the elderly is common. The majority of patients have so called senile pruritus and no clear cause is identified. This diagnosis would not be appropriate here as the patient has obvious erythema. An irritant dermatitis or drug eruption would, therefore, be a possible diagnosis. However, the changing clinical picture with the development of obvious blisters on inflamed skin strongly suggests that the clinical diagnosis is bullous pemphigoid, although a bullous adverse drug reaction would still have to be excluded.

The patient had a biopsy of the small, early, new blister, and both pathology and immunopathology were requested. The blister was subepidermal, and there was a linear band of IgG and also of C3 deposited at the dermal/epidermal junction (p. 234), confirming the clinical diagnosis of bullous pemphigoid.

Fig. 11.18 Staphylococcal scalded skin syndrome. Note superficial peeling which is due to the high level blistering.

Fig. 11.19 Papular urticaria. Crops of papules are seen most commonly on the lower legs.

Fig. 11.20 Urticaria pigmentosa. This 2-year-old child had three lesions which urticated on pressure and left surrounding pigmentation as seen here.

The patient was, therefore, commenced on prednisolone 40 mg orally per day, and over the next 7 days the erythema and blisters cleared. The steroid dose was reduced over 2 weeks to 10 mg a day, and over the following 4 months was discontinued completely.

Projects

1. Review the literature on epidermolysis bullosa produced by the patient support group Debra. Consider the implications of a diagnosis of any type of epidermolysis bullosa for a single parent in poor financial circumstances.

2. In several chapters the cutaneous problems caused by staphylococci have been considered. Draw all these together in a review of the skin diseases caused or aggravated by staphylococci.

Further reading

Wojnarowska, F. and Briggeman, R.A. (ed.) 1990. *Management of blistering diseases.* Chapman and Hall Medical, London.

Drug eruptions

- Themechanisms of cutaneous reactions to systemic drugs

- Commonly used systemic drugs in dermatology and their possible side-effects and interactions

- Adverse reactions to topical applications

There are three aspects of adverse drug reactions of particular importance to dermatologists. The first is that the commonest request for a dermatologist to visit in-patients in other hospital wards is to advise on suspected adverse reactions to systemically administered drugs. The second is the need for dermatologists to be aware of undesirable side effects and drug interactions of the systemic drugs commonly used in dermatology such as methotrexate, dapsone, and cyclosporin. The third is that topical therapy may also give rise to undesirable side-effects, as is the case with relatively potent topical steroid preparations. These are largely preventable.

Problem cases

Case 12.1

You are asked to see an elderly male with chronic obstructive airways disease on the respiratory wards. He has been admitted with an exacerbation due to infections and was started on an oral antibiotic 7 days ago. He is now erythrodermic with early blister formation on his trunk. He is also febrile and anuric. What is the likely diagnosis, the likely cause and the prognosis?

Case 12.2

A 20 year old college student home for the vacation consults you about a generalized macular rash and a general feeling of lethargy. She consulted the college medical officer about a sore throat last week and was given an antibiotic. She has not brought the remainder of the antibiotic capsules home with her and does not know the name of the antibiotic. What diagnosis does this presentation suggest and why?

The mechanisms of cutaneous reactions to systemic drugs

The majority of skin rashes induced by systemic medication are the result of immunological sensitization to the medicament. Ideally, it should be possible to classify them under Gell and Coombs' classic types of immunological reaction, namely:

- Type I   anaphylactic reactions
- Type II   cytotoxic reactions
- Type III   Arthus or immune complex mediated reactions
- Type IV   delayed hypersensitivity or cell-mediated reactions.

Key Points

It is important to obtain a complete history of medicaments, including any long-term drugs, 'natural remedies' and over-the-counter preparations that the patient may not consider important.

Fig. 12.1 Toxic erythema. This patient developed a morbilliform eruption 10 days after commencing a course of phenylbutazone.

Fig. 12.2 Mucous membrane and skin involvement in a child with drug-induced Stevens–Johnson syndrome.

In practice many adverse reactions are probably admixtures of two or more of these mechanisms.

History

The most important factor in establishing the likely precipitating agent in a suspected drug rash is a good history. However, the patients' notions of a 'drug' may be surprisingly variable, and laxatives, hypnotics, and simple analgesics are often regarded as part of a normal diet. Similarly, any medicament taken for a long period of time (for example a diuretic for the past year) seems scarcely to merit mention as patients tend to be keen to incriminate a newly added item. The most useful approach is to ask the patient to bring samples of all his or her pills and potions for inspection. A relative will often be invaluable in presenting a complete collection. A list from the family doctor is frequently incomplete for he may not be aware of patent medicines and other over-the-counter preparations.

Patients with rheumatological diseases seem relatively more susceptible to adverse drug reactions, probably due either to the nature of the medicaments or to inherently enhanced immunological responses. It should also be remembered that patients on multiple medication for general medical disorders may well have quite unrelated dermatological disorders. For example, scabies and asteatotic eczema may first make their appearance after hospital admission at a time when systemic medication is being considerably modified.

Clinical features

Table 12.1 lists drugs relatively frequently incriminated as causing drug eruptions, and Table 12.2 lists some of the cutaneous reaction patterns associated with drug reactions.

A common pattern of drug eruption is that of toxic erythema (Fig. 12.1). This is a widespread erythematous and morbilliform eruption which tends to affect the trunk more than the extremities. It appears 5–10 days after first introduction of the causative drug, but only 2–3 days after introduction if the drug has been given previously. Malaise, fever, and lymphadenopathy are common.

Other cutaneous reaction patterns associated with adverse drug reactions are erythema multiforme and its more severe form, the Stevens–Johnson syndrome (Fig. 12.2), erythema nodosum, vasculitic lesions and purpura, hair loss, pigmentation, exfoliative dermatitis, lichen planus-like eruptions, and urticaria (Figs 12.3–12.7).

Once a drug is strongly suspected it should be discontinued. If it has been the cause, the reaction can be expected to subside within the following 4–7 days. Confirmation by laboratory tests is not yet feasible as available *in vitro* immunological tests will yield both false-positive and false-negative results. No safe or satisfactory provocation test is available and challenge tests based on reintroduction of the drug are *not* recommended. Indeed, patients should be warned about the drugs incriminated and relevant notes made in case sheets or practice notes as subsequent exposure is likely to provoke more severe reactions.

Table 12.1.
Common causes of drug eruptions and likely patterns

Medicament	Pattern of eruption
Sulphonamides, pencillins	Morbilliform eruption, erythema multiforme, systemic lupus erythematosus
Phenylbutazone	Purpuric eruption
Beta-blockers	Psoriasiform
Barbiturates and tranquillizer overdosage	Blistering eruption of lower limbs
Pencillamine	Pemphigus-like eruption
Phenothiazines	Light-sensitive dermatosis
Antimalarials	Lichen planus-like eruption
Iodides and bromides	Acneiform eruption
Salicylates	Urticaria, angio-oedema

Fig. 12.3 Acute urticaria developing 4 hours after administration of systemic penicillin.

Table 12.2.

Cutaneous reaction patterns which may be due to drug reactions

Reaction pattern	Likely drugs
Toxic erythema	Antibodies (ampicillin), sulphonamides, barbiturates, antirheumatics
Erythema multiforme and Stevens–Johnson syndrome	Sulphonamides, antibiotics, antirheumatic drugs
Erythema nodosum	Sulphonamdies, contraceptive pill
Erythroderma	Antibiotics and antirheumatic drugs
Vasculitic and purpuric eruptions	Carbromal, phenytoin, indomethacin
Psoriasiform eruptions or aggravation of psoriasis	Beta-blockers, lithium
Very severe blistering eruption (toxic epidermal necrolysis)	Sulphonamides, allopurinol, phenylbutazone
Photosensitivity	Tetracyclines, phenothiazines
Alopecia	Coumarin anticoagulants, cytotoxics, antithyroid drugs
Acne, gingival hyperplasia	Phenytoin
SLE-like syndrome	Classically hydralazine. Also penicillin, sulphonamides, and, rarely, many others
Exfoliative dermatitis	Gold, isoniazid, phenylbutazone

The one exception to this rule is the morbilliform rash produced by ampicillin in patients with infectious mononucleosis (Fig. 12.8). For reasons which are not understood, this is a time-limited hypersensitivity and, once the infectious mononucleosis has resolved, the patient is unlikely to show an adverse reaction to ampicillin.

Penicillamine is used as a chelating agent and as an antirheumatic, and in a proportion of patients it causes a blistering eruption which is clinically, histologically, and immunologically identical to pemphigus vulgaris. The blistering eruption does not always subside after withdrawal of penicillamine.

Fig. 12.4 Purpuric lesions developing days after initial administration of oxyphenbutazone. The platelet count was normal.

Fig. 12.5 Pustular drug eruption due to bromide administration. Acneiform lesions are also seen.

In general medical wards adverse reactions to ingested drugs are by far the commonest dermatological problem. Review your prescribing habits and consider drug interactions carefully.

Treatment

Withdrawal of the likely drug is frequently all that is required, followed by careful instructions to the patient concerning future avoidance. In very severe anaphylactic reactions, emergency administration of subcutaneous adrenaline (0.5 ml of 1 in 1000 solution given slowly over 2–3 minutes) may be life-saving. Systemic antihistamines will relieve itch but there is little evidence that they accelerate spontaneous clearance of drug-induced lesions. Systemic corticosteroid administration may be of value, particularly in severe exfoliative dermatitis or

Fig. 12.6 Vesiculo-pustular drug eruption due to trimethoprim-sulphamethoxazole.

Fig. 12.7 Psoriasiform lesions developing for the first time 3 months after commencement of β-blocker therapy.

the Stevens–Johnson syndrome. An initial dose of parenteral hydrocortisone may be followed by oral prednisolone and withdrawn over a period of 7–10 days. Soothing topical therapy, such as simple calamine lotion or 1–2 per cent menthol in calamine cream, may also be helpful.

Key Points

Methotrexate	: drug interactions
Retinoids	: elevations of triglycerides
Cyclosporin	: renal toxicity
Dapsone	: haemolytic anaemia.

Commonly used systemic drugs in dermatology and their possible side-effects and interaction

Systemic drugs needed on occasion for difficult psoriasis include methotrexate, retinoids, and cyclosporin. With methotrexate the commonest problems are drug interactions, liver toxicity, and renal toxicity. The main problems associated with retinoid therapy are elevation of triglycerides and, most importantly,

Fig. 12.8 Morbilliform eruption caused by administration of ampicillin to a patient with infectious mononucleosis.

teratogenicity. Cyclosporin may be used in severe psoriasis, dermatitis, and experimentally in other conditions. Here the most serious potential problem is irreversible renal toxicity, and careful monitoring is essential.

Patients with dermatitis herpetiformis are commonly treated with dapsone. This can cause a haemolytic anaemia, commonest at the start of treatment, and patients should be carefully monitored during the first month of therapy. Patients on systemic steroids for dermatological problems should be monitored for hypertension glycosuria and excessive weight gain.

It is a good policy when starting any systemic drug in a patient who is already on other medication for unrelated problems to check possible drug interactions and, if necessary, amend prescribing plans. Local drug information centres, Martindales Pharmacopia, and the American Academy of Dermatology's Derminfonet are all useful sources of such information.

Adverse reactions to topical applications

Adverse reactions to topical applications are relatively common, especially to those containing antihistamines, anaesthetics, and antibiotics.

Antihistamines, if required, should only be given systemically as they are potent sensitizers when administered topically. The same applies to topical anaesthetics, and certain antibiotics—notably neomycin and sulphonamides—are equally troublesome. An added reason for avoiding their use topically is that, once sensitized, these patients will react subsequently to systemic as well as topical administration of the causative drug.

Adverse effects of topical corticosteroids

Sensibly used, topical steroids represent the most important advance in dermatological therapy in the past 30 years. However, as with any potent and effective form of therapy, they must be prescribed with care and common-sense,

Fig. 12.9 Striae on the axilla caused by topical steroid therapy.

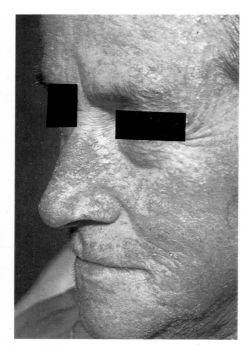

Fig. 12.10 Facial erythema and telangiectasia caused by application of potent topical steroid preparations.

bearing in mind that percutaneous absorption, particularly through inflamed and excoriated skin, can be significant. If large quantities of a potent steroid are applied continuously to damaged skin, all the classic side-effects associated with systemic steroid administration can occur, particularly in children. Much commoner, however, are the adverse effects on the skin itself. These are frequent and include a thin and fragile skin, spontaneous bruising, striae, and telangiectasia (Figs 12.9 and 12.10). The skin thinning, which is due to loss of dermal collagen, is reversible on withdrawal of the steroid, but striae and telangiectasia are permanent.

The speed of onset of such changes will depend on the site of application, the frequency of use, and the potency of the preparation. They develop rapidly in the warm humid microclimate of the body flexures.

Other complications of topical steroid therapy include tinea incognito, a term used to describe an atypical presentation of fungal infection on the skin due to unchecked growth of fungi on the steroid-treated skin. If simple scabies is not diagnosed or incorrectly treated with steroids the presentation may be confusing and atypical.

Sensitization to topical steroids leading to an allergic contact dermatitis is now well recognized, but may be difficult to identify in the early stages, as often topical steroids are prescribed for a dermatitis thought to be due to another cause. Tixocortol pivalate and budesonide are the commonest problems, and patch testing should be arranged if there is any suspicion.

The sensible approach to topical steroid usage is to prescribe the weakest effective preparation for as brief a spell as possible, and to review the patient regularly. This is particularly important in paediatric practice.

The choice of topical steroid preparation requires care. Table 12.3 divides a representative list of topical steroid preparations into very strong, strong, medium, and mild categories. Very much more extensive tables will be found in MIMS and the British National Formulary, and it is wise to consult these.

It is good practice only to prescribe preparations in the mild category for the face and flexures, and to avoid using the very strong preparations in children. It is possible to weaken a strong steroid by dilution, but the correct diluent must be used, otherwise all potency may be lost through the molecular change in the steroid molecule.

Discussion of problem cases

Case 12.1

The two most important conditions to consider here in the differential diagnosis are bullous pemphigoid and an adverse drug reaction. Patients with bullous pemphigoid generally are not unwell despite large blisters, so the fever and renal

Table 12.3.
Relative strengths of some topical steroid preparations

Very strong	Medium
Clobetasol propionate 0.05%	Hydrocortisone 17 butyrate 0/1% (Locoid)
	Clobetasone butyrate 0.05% (Eumovate)
(Dermovate, Removate)	Flurandrenolone 0.0125% (Haelan)
Strong	**Mild**
Bethamethasone 17-valerate 0.1% (Betnovate)	Hydrocortisone 0.1%, 1.0%, 2.5% (Efcortelan)
Beclomethaone dipropionate 0.25% (Propaderm)	Fluocinolone acetonide 0.01% (Synadone)
Betamethasone dipropionate Diprosone	Mild steroids are now available without prescription in the UK
Budesonide. Preferid	
Fluticasone propionate. Cutivate	

problems would be unusual. The clinical picture and the timing of its appearance both suggest that an adverse drug reaction to the antibiotic prescribed seven days earlier is the likely diagnosis. The features suggest toxic epidermal necrolysis which may be triggered by a number of antibiotics including septrin and penicillins. The antibiotic was withdrawn and the patient give systemic steroids. Despite this, his general condition deteriorated rapidly and he died three days later.

Review the literature on toxic epidermal necrolysis and its treatment with systemic steroids. What conclusions can you draw?

Case 12.2

This history is a very classic presentation of infectious mononucleosis (glandular fever). A young adult presents with general malaise and a sore throat for which penicillin is prescribed, and 4–7 days later a morbilliform eruption develops. The student had a positive monospot test. She slowly returned to normal energy levels over the next three months. Can she be given penicillins in the future?

Projects

1. Review the literature on amiodarone and cutaneous side-effects. What preventive action could you recommend if the drug was considered necessary?

2. Review the literature on beta blockers and psoriasiform eruptions. What conclusions can you draw?

Further reading

Breathnach, S.M. and Hintner, H. (1992). *Adverse drug reactions and the skin*. Blackwells, Oxford.

Bruinsma, W. (1995). *A guide to drug eruptions. The European file of side-effects in dermatology*. Free University, Amsterdam.

13

Cutaneous medicine

- Endocrine disorders: diabetes
  thyroid disfunction
  adrenal cortical disfunction
  acromegaly

- Gastrointestinal disorders: gluten-sensitive enteropathy
  malabsorption syndromes
  acrodermatitis enteropathica
  pyoderma gangrenosum
  Peutz–Jeghers syndrome
  Gardner's syndrome

- Other disorders: porphyria
  sarcoidosis
  hyperlipidaemias
  multiple neurofibromatosis
  Behçet's syndrome
  tuberous sclerosis
  nutritional disorders
  dermatitis artefacta

- Graft-versus host-disease—acute, chronic

- Investigation of pruritus

- Cutaneous manifestations of malignancy

Problem cases

Case 13.1

A patient consults you about non-painful red lesions, present on her shins for about 4 months. What would be the differential diagnosis in this case, what aspects of her medical history might be of relevance, and what treatments might be appropriate?

Case 13.2

A 38-year-old unemployed business man comes to see you because of blisters which have developed on his face during a recent spell of warm, sunny weather. He has been very depressed because of both family problems and inability to find employment and admits to drinking heavily. What is the differential diagnosis, what investigations might be appropriate, and what treatment is available?

Case 13.3

A healthy young woman whose only medication is the oral contraceptive comes to see you because of tender, red lumps on her lower legs which have been present for 5 days. What does this presentation suggest what are the possible causes and what investigations are indicated?

Case 13.4

A 14-year-old girl is brought to you by her mother for treatment of periungual warts. The girl attends a school for those with learning difficulties, and during the consultation, the mother who is very supportive asks also for help with acne like lesions around the girl's nose. On examination, the periungual lesions do not look like typical warts. What is the likely diagnosis in this case?

Introduction

In many systemic diseases the first signs are in the skin and thus they may alert the physician to a developing and possibly life-threatening condition. These diseases come under the general term of 'cutaneous medicine', an important 'link area' between dermatology and other specialties in which an alert dermatologist can, by careful history and examination, make a very valuable contribution.

Tables 13.1–13.3 list some of the commoner or more important diseases covered in this chapter. Inevitably, this is not exhaustive and the reader is referred to larger textbooks for a more comprehensive account.

Table 13.1.
Cutaneous manifestations of endocrine disease

Diabetes	Necrobiosis lipoidica (diabeticorum)
	Pruritus
	Fungal and bacterial skin infections
	Granuloma annulare
	Atherosclerosis and diabetic ischaemia
Hypothyroidism	Diffuse hair loss, coarse hair, broken hair
	Puffy oedema, xeroderma, pruritus
Hyperthyroidism	Hyperhidrosis
	Fine hair + hair loss, pruritus
	Pretibial myxoedema (usually associated with exophthalmos)
Cushing's syndrome	Acne vulgaris, hirsutism
	Cutaneous striae
	'Buffalo hump' obesity
Acromegaly	Soft tissue hypertrophy
	Seborrhoea
Addison's disease	Increased cutaneous pigmentation, especially intraoral

Cutaneous manifestations of endocrine disease

Diabetes

Patients with diabetes are at risk of a wide range of dermatological problems. Occasionally, the skin manifestations may be the first sign of diabetes, but more often they complicate pre-existing diabetes. Table 13.1 lists the commoner dermatological problems which may complicate diabetes.

Necrobiosis lipoidica diabeticorum (Fig. 13.1), is usually seen on the shins and may predate frank development of diabetes by several years. The individual lesions are shiny, atrophic, red or yellowish plaques with marked telangiectasia over their surface and a tendency to ulcerate. These ulcers may be very slow to heal. The severity of necrobiosis lipoidica is not directly related to the severity of the diabetes, nor does it improve with careful diabetic control.

Fig. 13.1 Necrobiosis lipoidica. Firm, reddish-yellow plaques are seen on the shins.

Treatment is unsatisfactory, but protection from trauma and resultant skin damage are important. Intralesional injections of a steroid such as triamcinolone acetonide may be initially beneficial in some cases.

Many patients with diabetes complain of pruritus. This is sometimes but not always related to poor control of diabetes. Pruritus vulvae is relatively common in female diabetics, and urine should always be checked for glycosuria in a patient first presenting with this problem. Those with diabetes are particularly prone to bacterial and fungal skin infections, and again diabetes should be excluded in any stubborn or unusually florid infection of this type.

Granuloma annulare is found more commonly on the skin of diabetics than by chance (Fig. 13.2). The condition is commoner in children than in adults, and it would appear to be more frequently associated with diabetes when it occurs in

Key Points

Granuloma annulare can be misdiagnosed as a fungal infection.

Fig. 13.2 Granuloma annulare on a typical site, the dorsum of the hand.

Fig. 13.3 Pretibial myxoedema. Raised, reddish plaques and nodules are seen on the shins.

adults. The lesions are erythematous and circular with a well- marked, raised, palpable lateral border. The hands and feet are most commonly affected. The lesions are frequently multiple and tend to clear spontaneously after 3–6 months or longer. Occasionally, trauma, such as a diagnostic biopsy, appears to stimulate spontaneous clearance in the remainder of the lesion.

Secondary trophic change from diabetic ischaemia and atherosclerosis is a less specific, but accepted association, and if these changes are present diabetic gangrene is a very real hazard of inexpert chiropody or minor trauma.

Thyroid dysfunction

Abnormal hair growth is common in thyroid disease. Classically, in myxoedema the scalp hair is sparse, coarse, and brittle and the outer part of the eyebrows is lost, while in **hyperthyroidism** there is fine scalp hair, and sometimes associated alopecia.

Pretibial myxoedema is seen mainly after successful treatment of hyperthyroidism, especially when there are also ophthalmological complications. Clinically, there are asymptomatic, raised, red nodules and, although the name suggests that they are found chiefly on the shins (Fig. 13.3), they are also seen around the ankle and on the dorsum of the foot. Histological examination shows oedema and mucin. These patients have high levels of long acting thyroid stimulating hormone (LATS).

Topical corticosteroid preparations may be of some benefit but, in general, these lesions are resistant to any type of treatment.

Adrenal cortical hyperfunction—Cushing's disease

This may present with acne vulgaris, seborrhoea, and hirsutism. Cutaneous striae may develop with great rapidity and be associated with 'buffalo hump' type of obesity. If due to endogenous steroids, a search for enlarged adrenals, excessive production from the adrenals, or an adrenal tumour should be carried out. However a high proportion of patients with cutaneous lesions suggestive of Cushing's disease have these as a secondary phenomenon due to oral steroid administration for another disease, and it may be necessary to continue oral steroid therapy.

Adrenal cortical hypofunction—Addison's disease

Adrenal cortical hypofunction may be associated with a striking increase in melanin pigmentation, particularly on mucous membranes and sites of friction (Fig. 13.4). This is a result of melanocyte stimulation by raised circulating levels of ACTH.

Fig. 13.4 Intraoral melanin pigmentation seen in Addison's disease.

Acromegaly

This condition is associated with acne, seborrhoea, and soft tissue hypertrophy (Fig. 13.5). It is can easily be confused initially with adrenal hyperfunction.

Cutaneous associations of gastrointestinal disease

Gluten-sensitive enteropathy

Gluten-sensitive enteropathy is common in dermatitis herpetiformis and has already been discussed (p. 235).

Malabsorption syndromes

These may lead to a secondary dermatosis in which there are moist, eczematous skin lesions chiefly in the flexures. These may have a psoriasiform appearance and a small proportion of patients may have deficiencies of trace metals, such as zinc.

Acrodermatitis enteropathica

Acrodermatitis enteropathica is a genetically determined disorder due to grossly defective zinc absorption. It is frequently first seen when the infant is being weaned off breast milk and presents as erythematous, raw, and pustular areas around the mouth, anus, fingers, and toes. Severe diarrhoea is common, and if the condition is not recognized and treated, hair and nails will be shed. Oral zinc supplements bring about dramatic and rapid improvement, and must be continued for many years, possibly for life.

A similar condition is seen in patients receiving total parenteral nutrition or elemental diets in which zinc is lacking. Onset can be very rapid, but once the diagnosis is made and zinc supplements administered, the lesions clear equally rapidly.

Fig. 13.5 Acromegaly. Note soft tissue hypertrophy, acne, and seborrhoea.

Table 13.2.

Commoner dermatological associations with gastrointestinal disease

Dermatitis herpetiformis	Gluten-sensitive enteropathy
Flexural eczematous eruptions	Malabsorption
	Mild zinc deficiency states
Acrodermatitis enteropathica	Defective zinc absorption
Peutz–Jeghers syndrome	Polyps of small intestine
Gardner's syndrome	Polyps of large intestine
Pyoderma gangrenosum	Ulcerative colitis, Crohn's disease, rheumatoid arthritis
Perineal ulceration and skin tags; sinus formation	Crohn's disease

Pyoderma gangrenosum

Pyoderma gangrenosum (p. 181) may precede the development of frank gastrointestinal symptoms in both ulcerative colitis and Crohn's disease. Patients with Crohn's disease also tend to have multiple perianal skin tags, ulcers, and fistulae, and occasionally severe oral ulceration. Pyoderma gangrenosum is also associated with rheumatoid arthritis and Still's disease.

Peutz–Jeghers syndrome

The Peutz–Jeghers syndrome consists of freckle-like pigmentation on and around the lips, and polyposis of the gastrointestinal tract, particularly the small bowel. Intussusception may develop, but the polyps are rarely premalignant (Fig. 13.6).

Photosensitivity

Unusual cutaneous reactions to natural sunlight may be part of a systemic disease or an isolated finding. Some of the commoner causes are lupus erythematosus, rosacea, and porphyria. A number of drugs may also cause a photosensitive eruption. These include non-steroid anti-inflammatories, thiazide diuretics, antibiotics, and anti-arrhythmics such as amiodarone. It is particularly important to warn elderly patients of possible photosensitivity prior to a holiday or prolonged winter break in a sunnier climate than usual.

Fig. 13.6 Peutz–Jeghers syndrome. Macular melanin pigmentation is seen on and around the lips

Table 13.3.
Cutaneous features of other systemic disease

Porphyria	Photosensitivity
	Skin fragility, blister formation
	Hypertrichosis, pigmentation
Sarcoidosis	Blue-red subcutaneous nodules
	Lupus pernio
	'Scar' sarcoid
Hyperlipidaemias	Xanthomata–tendinous, tuberous, and eruptive
Neurofibromatosis	Multiple cutaneous neurofibromata
	Freckling and *café au lait* spots
Tuberous sclerosis	'Adenoma sebaceum' (perifollicular fibromata)
	Periungual fibromata
	Shagreen patches
Pellagra (nicotinic acid deficiency)	'Diarrhoea, dermatitis and dementia'
	Erythema after sunlight exposure
Scurvy (vitamin C deficiency)	Bleeding gums, purpura, poor wound healing

Fig. 13.7 Cutaneous hepatic porphyria. Hyperpigmentation and hypertrichosis are present.

Fig. 13.8 Polymorphic light eruptions. Typical appearance in early spring of acute facial eruption on 13-year-old girl.

Other disorders

Porphyria

The porphyrias frequently present with cutaneous signs and symptoms. **Porphyria cutanea tarda** is most likely to present to the dermatologist, and is characterized by photosensitivity, skin fragility, subepidermal blister formation, and hyperpigmentation and hypertrichosis of sun-exposed skin (Fig. 13.7). There is usually a history of underlying liver damage, due most commonly to excessive alcohol intake. The diagnosis can be confirmed by demonstrating grossly elevated levels of urinary uroporphyrins. Elevated levels of serum iron are a feature and venesection to reduce this will alleviate symptoms. A variety of drugs aggravate the condition and the patient should be given written instructions on avoidance of these.

Other much rarer forms of porphyria may present to dermatologists. In **erythropoietic protoporphyria** very brief exposure to sunlight may cause itch, pain, and oedema. Pitted scars tend to develop on facial skin. Elevated erythrocyte and plasma protoporphyrin levels confirm the diagnosis. Topical sun-screens, particularly preparations which give physical protection with titanium dioxide, will give symptomatic relief.

Sunscreens can be divided into those which give physical protection by deflecting UV rays and chemical protection which absorbs UV. Physical sunscreens contain zinc or titanium dioxide and although perhaps less cosmetically acceptable they are very effective.

Polymorphic light eruption

Polymorphic light eruption is a common photosensitive disorder, seen most often in young females. Patients are particularly sensitive to long wave UV in the 320–360 nm range of the spectrum (UVA), and typically present in the early spring with itchy papules on the face and hands (Fig. 13.8). There appears to be some hardening as the rash becomes less troublesome as the season advances, but tends to recur in the following spring. Monochromator photosensitivity testing will confirm the diagnosis.

Patients can be treated by slow desensitization, using a UVA source, or can be advised to use a broad spectrum sunscreen.

Sarcoidosis

Sarcoidosis frequently presents with cutaneous lesions. The basic pathological process is non-caseating granuloma formation in a variety of sites. The cause is not yet known, but it may be significant that sarcoidosis is much commoner in countries where tuberculosis has been well controlled. The commonest dermatological presentation of sarcoidosis is **erythema nodosum** and an appearance on chest X-ray of hilar lymphadenopathy.

Other cutaneous signs of sarcoid are **lupus pernio** (Fig. 13.9)—blue-red nodules on the nose, face, and hands—and **scar sarcoid**—the development of sarcoid granulomas in scars.

The **Kveim test** can be used to confirm the diagnosis. Kveim antigen is injected intradermally, and 6 weeks later the site is biopsied and examined carefully for evidence of granuloma formation. Practical details are important if a valid result of this test is to be obtained: the antigen must be injected intradermally, not subcutaneously; the syringe used should be glass, not disposable plastic which may be lubricated with a granuloma-producing material; and the injection site must be marked accurately with reference to bony landmarks. Reference to moles or freckles can cause confusion. Most patients with sarcoid have elevated levels of angiotensin converting enzyme but this is not a finding specific to sarcoid. Treatment of sarcoid is unsatisfactory. Patients with erythema nodosum and hilar adenopathy usually have a self-limiting condition, but lupus pernio tends to persist and can be very disfiguring. Low dose, alternate day systemic steroids may be helpful.

Hyperlipidaemias

The hyperlipidaemias may present or be associated with **xanthelasmata** and **xanthomata**. Xanthelasmata are white or yellow plaques of lipid deposited in the periorbital skin. The majority of these are not associated with hyperlipaemic states and are of cosmetic importance only, but in 10–20 per cent of cases fasting lipids will be elevated. An arcus senilis may also be seen. Simple xanthelasma should be treated, if necessary, by excision or destruction with trichloracetic acid.

Most **cutaneous xanthomata** are eruptive, tendinous, or tuberous (Fig. 13.10). The rare variant of **plane xanthoma** may resemble plane warts and may be associated with paraproteinaemia. Eruptive lesions occur on any body site and have an inflammatory halo. Tendinous lesions are most commonly seen over the Achilles tendon or on the dorsa of the hands, and tuberous lesions, which may be very large and bizarre in shape, tend to be prominent around knees and elbows. Xanthomata may be a pointer either to a primary hyperlipaemic state due to a genetic abnormality or to a secondary hyperlipaemic state due to renal, hepatic, endocrine, or pancreatic disease. The hyperlipaemias are classified according to relative proportions on serum electrophoresis of α-lipoprotein, pre-β-lipoprotein, β-lipoprotein, and chylomicrons. Treatment will vary according to the type of hyperlipoproteinaemia identified, and may include dietary restriction of fat and carbohydrate, possibly with additional systemic therapy such as bezafibrate or pravastatin.

Multiple neurofibromatosis (von Recklinghausen's disease)

This genodermatosis is inherited as an autosomal dominant trait, so a positive family history is usually present. The majority of patients who have cutaneous features of neurofibromatosis have neurofibromatosis type 1(NF1). The NF1 gene has been identified, and is a very large gene on chromosome 17q11.2.

The cutaneous features include macular hyperpigmentation (*café au lait* patches), neurofibromata, and multiple skin tags (**molluscum fibrosum**). These are soft, sessile, pink lesions which may be extremely numerous and disfiguring (Fig. 13.11). The pigmentary changes may be relatively mild, but the presence of

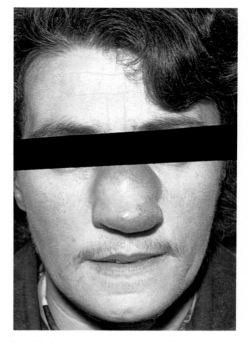

Fig. 13.9 Lupus pernio seen in sarcoidosis.

Fig. 13.10 Tuberous xanthomata. This patient had a normal lipoprotein profile.

Fig. 13.11 Multiple molluscum fibrosum of von Recklinghausen's disease.

even a few macular pigmented lesions in the axillary vaults is regarded by some workers as pathognomonic. Forty per cent of sufferers may develop neurological complications such as acoustic neuroma or optic nerve glioma and careful neurological examination at presentation, and thereafter, is therefore important. Sarcomatous change within such a tumour is reported.

Behçet's syndrome

The cardinal features of this condition are severe and persistent oral and genital ulceration, iritis, and arthropathy (Fig. 13.12). A viral aetiology is postulated. Involvement of the central nervous system may result in a pattern very similar to disseminated sclerosis. An interesting dermatological feature is 'hyperergy', that is the tendency of sterile blisters to develop at venepuncture sites. Behçet's syn-

Fig. 13.12 Behçet's syndrome. Severe oral ulcers are seen. Genital ulcers and iritis were also present.

drome will come into the differential diagnosis of severe persistent blistering on mucosal surfaces. The diagnosis will be confirmed by excluding other causes, and by identifying non-cutaneous features of Behçet's. Treatment is difficult. Systemic steroids or cyclosporin may help some cases.

Tuberous sclerosis (epiloia, Bourneville's disease)

Tuberous sclerosis is inherited by autosomal dominant transmission, but may not first present until puberty or later. The gene is situated on chromosome 9q34.

Tuberous sclerosis comprises the triad of cutaneous abnormalities, mental retardation, and seizures. There are four main types of skin lesions:

- **periungual fibromata**—multiple, hypertrophic nodules around the nails which may look rather like viral warts (Fig. 13.13);

- **shagreen patches**—normal-coloured plaques on the trunk which have a firmer texture than normal skin;

- **adenoma sebaceum**—this term is pathologically incorrect as these lesions are in fact **perivascular fibromata** and are raised, red papules on the face, mainly around the nose (Fig. 13.14);

- **ash-leaf hypopigmentation**—this is well demonstrated under Wood's light as multiple, oval areas of hypopigmentation and may be the earliest sign of the disorder.

The individual prognosis varies with the degree of mental retardation and neurological involvement. Treatment of the perivascular fibromata with diathermy surgery or laser therapy will produce a considerable cosmetic improvement.

Key Points

It is possible to mistake adenoma sebaceum of tuberous sclerosis for acne.

Fig. 13.13 Periungual fibroma in a child with tuberous sclerosis. Note wart-like lesions between nail and nail fold.

Fig. 13.14 Adenoma sebaceum (perifollicular fibroma) of tuberous sclerosis.

Nutritional deficiency disorders

A variety of relative nutritional disorders may present with cutaneous lesions in the absence of frank malnutrition.

Scurvy: Hypovitaminosis C, even frank scurvy, is seen in elderly people on a self-imposed 'tea and toast' diet. Their bleeding gums, easy bruising, and even frank purpura may all be dismissed as 'age changes'. In such cases, low levels of leucocyte ascorbic acid will confirm the diagnosis and oral vitamin C supplements will be curative.

Pellagra: This is due to nicotinic acid deficiency. It is rare, and presents with dermatitis, diarrhoea, and dementia. The dermatitis affects sun-exposed sites and consists of scaly erythema with a clear-cut, raised lateral margin, and subsequent hyperpigmentation. This is sometimes called Casals collar or Casal's necklace. The antituberculous drug INAH can cause the same syndrome. Nicotinic acid replacement is rapidly curative.

Kwashiorkor: In kwashiorkor (protein malnutrition) the affected infant's skin is dry, with a glazed erythematous eruption, and the hair is dry, brittle, and hypopigmented. Oedema and ascites may also be present.

Dermatitis artefacta (factitial dermatitis), dermatological Munchausen's disease

Definition

Bizarre lesions on any body site deliberately initiated or aggravated by the patient.

Incidence and aetiology

This condition is rare, and commoner in women than in men. In some cases 'dermatological malingering' or self-induced aggravation of pre-existing lesions

Key Points

Dermatitis artefacta is rare but should be considered in bizarre lesions, particularly on an exposed site.

may be related to claims for industrial compensation, but in the majority no obvious motive is identified. Many patients are withdrawn, solitary individuals and consultation with medical attendants is one of their few social contacts. Clearly, complicated psychological motives, and at times frank psychoses, are involved in the aetiology of this group of disorders, but recognition of this and appropriate referral is not always accompanied by disappearance of lesions.

Clinical features

These are varied and diverse. The condition should be considered in any bizarre skin lesion, particularly if it is on an exposed site and is an unusual angular or geometric shape (Fig. 13.15). Application of caustic liquids to the skin will cause erythema to develop on the site of drips or splashes from the applicator. Material may be injected into the skin, and finger-nails and hair may be damaged or even removed. Important pointers are an inappropriate interest in the lesions with relative lack of real concern, and persistence or extension of the lesions if treated as an out-patient. In contrast, hospital admission is often accompanied by rapid healing of the lesions.

Treatment

This is difficult. Direct confrontation will usually result in angry denial and failure to keep return appointments. A complicated degree of collusion may exist between the patient and the patient's relatives so that they too may react in this manner to a direct statement that the lesions are self-provoked. Similarly, referral for psychiatric consultation may be the signal for the patient to remove him/herself to the care of another dermatologist. In general, treatment and, on occasion, cessation of self-mutilation becomes possible when the dermatologist establishes a degree of rapport with the patient and it is understood, but not frankly stated, that both parties know how the lesions are produced. Collaborative treatment with a sympathetic psychiatrist may be beneficial, but much can be achieved by emotional support. The lesions will clear speedily if occlusive dressings and bandaging are used, but tend to recur on other body sites.

Cutaneous graft-versus-host disease

This is now much less common than 5 years ago as a result of pre-conditioning of bone marrow prior to infusion into the recipient.

Although there is some overlap, graft-versus-host disease has two relatively distinct clinical presentations. These are early onset graft-versus-host disease appearing within 100 days of marrow transplant, and late or chronic graft-versus-host disease appearing after the 100-day period.

Acute graft-versus-host disease

Affected patients usually have the triad of fever, diarrhoea, and a skin rash. This is commonly seen 7–10 days after the marrow graft at a time when the patient has been on multiple drug therapy. Consequently, the rash, which may be

Fig. 13.15 Dermatitis artefacta. Note striking bizarre lesions on patient's trunk.

Fig. 13.16 Acute graft versus host disease. Note palmar erythema.

transient, may very easily be confused with a drug eruption. The rash of graft-versus-host disease at this stage is maculopapular and tends to involve the trunk, the palms (Fig. 13.16), the soles, and the oral mucous membranes. These latter three sites may be of some value in differentiating the rash from a drug eruption. A skin biopsy taken at this point in time will show a lichenoid tissue reaction in the skin with liquefaction degeneration of the basement membrane and will frequently show the histological sign of 'satellite cell necrosis'. This describes the pattern within the epidermis of a lymphocyte in contact with an apparently necrotic keratinocyte. It is not totally specific for graft-versus-host disease, but its presence will add weight to the diagnosis.

Chronic graft-versus-host disease

The onset of this form of graft-versus-host disease is usually more insidious. Patients may first notice a darkening of their normal skin colour, followed by a tightening and sclerosis of the skin causing immobility and contractures. Hair and nails may be shed, and the overall picture resembles that of systemic sclerosis. A skin biopsy taken from this type of graft-versus-host disease will show very gross thickening of the dermal collagen.

Treatment

Treatment of either type of graft-versus-host disease is difficult, but the acute phase may respond to high-dose oral steroid therapy.

The investigation of pruritus

A number of systemic disease states may present with persistent and severe pruritus of clinically normal skin. Patients are usually elderly and may complain bitterly of sleep loss due to clamant itch. However great the temptation to dismiss the condition as 'simple pruritus' or even 'neurotic excoriation', it is important to take a careful history and carry out appropriate investigations to exclude both simple remediable exogenous causes and more serious precipitating factors.

History-taking must include details of occupational exposure to possible causative agents (for example irritant dermatitis due to fibreglass), and also details of recreational and domestic agents. Take a careful family and contact history, and remember that scabies in the well washed can be very atypical. A careful history of topical and systemic drugs used currently and in the recent past is also essential. Well-demarcated, localized pruritus may be exogenous, but generalized itch is more likely to be due to a systemic cause.

A list of the commoner systemic associations of severe, generalized pruritus is given in Table 13.4. Diabetes, primary biliary cirrhosis, and polycythaemia are frequent associations.

After obtaining a full history, appropriate investigations should be initiated. Initial screening tests should include a full blood count, chest X-ray, serum urea, electrolytes and cholesterol, serum iron and TIBC levels, liver enzymes, thyroid function studies, and an autoantibody screen. More specialized, subsequent investigation will depend on the history and results of this screening procedure. If all results are negative, a diagnosis of idiopathic or 'senile' pruritus may be justified. Relief from pruritus in this condition may be obtained by vigorously treating the dry skin (xerosis, *eczema craquelé*) which is frequently present. The prescription of lubricant bath oils and substitution of emulsifying ointment BP or liquid paraffin 50 per cent in white soft paraffin in place of soap may be curative.

Table 13.4.
Some of the commoner systemic disease associations with cutaneous pruritus

Diabetes mellitus

Thyroid dysfunction (hypo- and hyperthyroidism)

Hepatic disease

Primary biliary cirrhosis

Chronic renal failure: itch may be present despite regular dialysis and normal blood urea

Polycythaemia

Haemochromatosis

Lymphoma

Hodgkin's disease

Neurological disorders, e.g. tabes dorsalis

Parasitosis

Drug addiction and abuse

Systemic antihistamines may give some relief but may also cause confusion in the elderly and should therefore be used with caution.

In **pruritus ani** and **pruritus vulvae** it is important to exclude easily remediable infections such as candidosis, trichomonal vaginitis, and thread-worms. Women should be examined carefully for the presence of lichen sclerosis et atrophicus (p. 160), although here both itch and pain are the usual symptoms. The urine should be tested for sugar to exclude occult diabetes. In a high proportion, however, no obvious precipitating cause will be identified. Many of these patients are relatively obsessional, rather tense individuals whose symptoms flare at times of domestic or occupational stress. Both psychosomatic and psychosexual explanations have been offered for their symptoms.

Treatment should include advice on the avoidance of proprietary local anaesthetic preparations which can cause allergic contact dermatitis. Weak topical steroid/antibiotic combinations may offer some relief. Systemic antihistamines and antidepressants may be of some value, but the condition tends to recur.

Cutaneous manifestations of systemic malignancy

An interesting group of cutaneous lesions are those associated with internal malignancy. This group of lesions may indeed be the pointer to a systemic neoplasm which has not yet been recognized, and is therefore an important area of collaboration between the dermatologist and the general physician or internist. The list of skin conditions in this category can be very long indeed and it is important to remember that in some cases solid epidemiological evidence of the association is lacking. Many of these cutaneous problems are seen predominantly in the elderly who have a high incidence of all types of malignancy. Nevertheless, the conditions listed below should prompt the thought that there may also be an occult and possibly curable malignancy present.

Acanthosis nigricans

This rare condition, which may be associated with malignancy or gross obesity, is characterized by hyperpigmentation and hyperkeratosis, most marked in the body flexures. The commonest association is with gastrointestinal malignancies (Fig. 13.17).

Dermatomyositis

This condition has already been discussed (p. 161). Ten to twenty-five per cent of adult-onset dermatomyositis have been reported to be associated with an occult malignancy involving any body site. The dermatomyositis may precede the development of the malignancy by months or even years. Removal of the tumour may result in clearance of the dermatomyositis.

Glucagonoma (necrolytic migratory erythema)

These patients present with a raw, painful tongue, and superficial erosions and blisters on the face, buttocks, thighs, and abdomen. Diabetes is present and the

Fig. 13.17 Acanthosis nigricans of the inner thigh. This patient had a carcinoma of stomach.

malignancy is generally a glucagon-secreting tumour of the pancreatic islet cells. Removal of the tumour will result in dramatic clearance of the skin lesions.

Acquired ichthyosis

The development of excessively dry and scaly skin in elderly patients may herald the development of Hodgkin's disease, non-Hodgkin's lymphoma, or a solid tumour.

Bowen's disease

A small proportion of patients with Bowen's carcinoma *in situ* of the skin (p. 289) will also have an unrelated systemic neoplasm.

Cowden's disease (multiple hamartoma syndrome)

This condition is a marker for breast and thyroid malignancies. Although rare, it is important, as the association with malignancy is so strong. Patients develop multiple papules and papillomata on the face, hands, and forearms and also have papules and a cobblestone appearance on the mucous membranes. Neural abnormalities may also be present.

Paraneoplastic acrokeratosis (Bazex syndrome)

Patients with this rare condition develop psoriasiform plaques on the hands, feet, and face. There is thickening of the palmar and plantar skin, and the nails may become dystrophic and break easily. All reported cases of the condition to date have had a malignancy of the pharynx or larynx.

Gardner's syndrome

This syndrome is characterized by sebaceous and epidermal cysts, skeletal abnormalities, and polyposis coli. The polyps, which may be asymptomatic, mainly involve the large bowel and malignant change in these polyps is recorded in about one-third of cases.

Other associations

Other rare associations between cutaneous lesions and systemic malignancy include severe herpes zoster and erythema gyratum repens (a pattern of cutaneous erythema resembling wood grain which rapidly changes shape on the skin), and the sudden appearance of profuse growth of lanugo hair or of multiple basal cell papillomata. Individual case reports associate severe bullous pemphigoid with concomitant systemic malignancy, but this may be a chance association of two conditions both commoner in elderly people.

Discussion of problem cases

Case 13.1

Red areas on the shins alone suggests erythema nodosum, pretibial myxoedema, or necrobiosis lipoidica. In this case, the duration and lack of pain do not make erythema nodosum likely. A careful history should be taken of symptoms or past treatment related to either thyroid problems or diabetes. The patient had no thyroid related problems, but did have a strong family history of insulin dependent diabetes. A biopsy confirmed the presence of palisading granulomas typical of necrobiosis lipoidica. The lesions responded slightly to topical steroid application, and three years later the patient developed frank diabetes.

This case illustrates the fact that necrobiosis lipoidica can precede development of diabetes.

Case 13.2

The differential diagnosis of blisters in an adult include a bullous adverse drug reaction, bullous pemphigoid, and problems associated with systemic disease including porphyria. The patient was on no possibly relevant drugs, and the distribution of the blisters was not typical of pemphigoid. The history of excess alcohol and the fact that the blisters are all on sun exposed sites suggests cutaneous hepatic porphyria. Blood porphyrin levels confirmed this clinical diagnosis, and it was also noted that the patient had a very high serum iron. Other cutaneous feature noted were hypertrichosis around the temples, and poor healing after minor trauma.

The patient was counselled on restricting alcohol intake, and had a pint of blood removed weekly for six weeks. The blisters cleared on this routine and did not recur.

Case 13.3

The rapid onset of painful nodules confined only to the shins suggests a diagnosis of erythema nodosum. A biopsy will confirm this. Erythema nodosum is, however, a tissue reaction pattern which may be caused by a wide range of precipitating agents which will need to be sought in this case. Drugs are a common cause of erythema nodosum and the oral contraceptive could be responsible, but other causes should first be excluded.

On chest X-ray, the young woman was found to have hilar adenopathy. The combination of hilar adenopathy and erythema nodosum is the commonest pattern of presentation of sarcoidosis. She also had a raised serum angiotensin converting enzyme level, and on this basis a diagnosis of sarcoidosis was made.

With no treatment other than rest, the lesions of erythema nodosum resolved over the following 6 weeks, and 6 months later her chest X-ray was normal.

Case 13.4

Unusual periungual lesions, learning difficulties and a facial eruption around the nasolabial folds should alert you to the possibility of tuberous sclerosis. It is not unusual for the diagnosis to be made after the periungual fibromata have been mistaken for warts but have not responded to treatment. A large proportion of patients with tuberous sclerosis appear to have spontaneous mutations of the TS gene as there is a negative family history.

In this girl's case the diagnosis was confirmed by cerebral CT. She also had shagreen patches on her trunk. Her parents were informed of the diagnosis, counselled on the likely progression,and given information about the Tuberous Sclerosis Association.

Projects

1. Review the cutaneous problems associated with gastrointestinal disease. Try to quantitate this by relating the prevalence of a disease such as Crohn's disease to the frequency with which you find reports of apparently associated cutaneous problems in the literature. How accurate do you think such a quantitiation might be? Are you likely to arrive at an underestimate or an overestimate and why?

2. Review the literature on the genetics of neurofibromatosis and the clinical variations associated with the different genetic abnormalities.

Further reading

Callen, J.P., Jorizzo, J., Greer, K., Penneys, N., Piette, W., and Zone, J.Z. (1988). *Dermatological signs of internal disease*. W.B. Saunders, Philadelphia.

14

Benign and malignant skin tumours

- Benign: Basal cell papillomas or seborrhoeic keratoses
  Epidermal naevi
  Pyogenic granuloma
  Histiocytoma
  Skin appendage tumours

- Potentially premalignant: Actinic keratoses
  Bowen's disease
  Keratoacanthoma

- Malignant: Squamous cell carcinoma
  Xeroderma pigmentosum
  Basal cell carcinoma
  Basal cell naevus (Gorlin's) syndrome
  Malignant melanoma
  Histiocytosis X
  Merkel cell tumour
  Kaposi's sarcoma

- Cutaneous lymphoma (Mycosis fungoids)

- Metastases to the skin from other sites.

Problem cases

Case 14.1

Last week there was a 40 minute television documentary from Australia on a young man dying of melanoma which has aroused a lot of additional publicity. This week you have three patients who have seen the documentary and who are concerned.

The first is an elderly lady who lives alone and who is very worried about several fairly large, growing lesions on her back. She does not know how long they have been there, but tells you that from time to time parts of the lesions crumble off.

The second is a young man brought to you by his wife. He has had a congenital melanocytic naevus, 5 cm in largest diameter, on his thigh since birth but over the past 2 years it has developed several central areas of dark brown to black pigmentation.

The third is a woman in her late twenties who is concerned about an irregular pigmented lesion on her upper arm present and growing for about a year. It has an irregular outline, and has areas of tan and blue-black coloration.

What action do you take in each of these three situations?

Case 14.2

An elderly male consults you about a solitary, scaling, crusting lesion over his left scapula. He has no idea how long it has been present. He is also receiving treatment for prostate cancer. What is the differential diagnosis here, what is the most likely diagnosis, and what action do you take?

Case 14.3

A female missionary in her 50s consults you about diffuse hair loss. In the course of the consultation you notice a translucent, nodular about 1 cm across below her left eye. What action do you take?

Case 14.4

The professional at the local golf club consults you about irritable, crusting lesions on his scalp. He has extensive male pattern baldness, but when younger was red haired. What is the likely diagnosis here and what is an appropriate management plan?

Introduction

Benign epidermal tumours and naevi arising from either keratinocytes or melanocytes are extremely common and increase in prevalence with age, particularly on white skin. Benign tumours or naevi arising from the Langerhans cell or Merkel cell have not yet been identified.

There is also a wide range of benign lesions arising from dermal cells, and a very wide, but relatively rare, range of benign or only locally expansile tumours arising from cells involved in the skin appendages. It is extremely useful to be able to identify clinically at least the commoner of these benign cutaneous lesions, as many need no treatment other than to reassure the patient. Melanocytic naevi have already been discussed on page 204.

There is a smaller range of benign tumours or naevi which have the capacity for malignant transformation, and here again clinical recognition is useful, but often surgical removal is needed to confirm a clinical diagnosis. If not, surveillance may be necessary.

Malignant tumours arising from the epidermal keratinocyte—the basal and squamous cell carcinomas—are the commonest malignancies of all, but are often omitted from cancer registration returns because of the belief that they are very rarely fatal. While this is in general true, the workload generated in removing these non-melanomas skin cancers is considerable, especially in a country such as Australia where a high proportion of white skinned individuals are exposed to long hours of natural sunlight.

The cutaneous malignancy responsible for the majority of skin cancer related deaths is the malignant melanoma, arising from the epidermal melanocyte. Malignant melanoma is of particular current interest because of its rapidly increasing incidence in all parts of the world, and because of the fact that it affects relatively young adults in the third and fourth decades, thus resulting in a high number of years of potential lost life for every melanoma death.

Malignant tumours also arise in the dermis, and at present the malignancy of most interest in this category is Kaposi's sarcoma, arising from the dermal vasculature. A subset of patients who develop Kaposi's sarcoma have AIDS, but there are also other at risk groups.

Cutaneous lymphoma is relatively rare, but may at times come into the differential diagnosis of psoriasis.

Finally, it should be remembered that the epidermis, and more often the dermis, can be the site of metastatic spread from primary tumours arising in other parts of the body.

Key Points

Benign tumours are common.

Factors predisposing to cutaneous malignancy

Both genetic and environmental factors influence the development of cutaneous malignancy.

The two genodermatoses predisposing to cutaneous malignancy are xeroderma pigmentosum (p. 292), associated with defective, unscheduled DNA repair which predisposes to all types of cutaneous malignancy but especially squamous cell carcinoma, and Gorlin's syndrome or the basal cell naevus syndrome which predisposes to basal cell carcinoma (p. 294).

The major environmental factor currently recognized as predisposing to skin cancer is excessive exposure of pale skin to natural ultraviolet radiation. Prolonged exposure to ultraviolet radiation in the UVB (280–320 nm) part of the spectrum is carcinogenic in man, and a clear quantitative, linear relationship exists between UVB exposure of Caucasian skin and the incidence of squamous carcinoma. The evidence for sunlight in general, and UVB in particular, influencing the incidence of cutaneous malignant melanoma is also strong, but the relationship here is not so clear-cut as with squamous carcinoma. Despite this, there is a clear increase in incidence of melanoma in the south of Norway by comparison with the north and the highest incidence of melanoma recorded in the world is among the white population of Queensland, Australia.

Incidence figures for both malignant melanoma and squamous carcinoma in black- and white-skinned populations in the same geographic area show a very much lower figure for black populations, suggesting that melanin plays a significant role in protecting against ultraviolet-induced carcinogenesis.

Case control studies from many parts of the world in the past decade have clearly indicated that for both melanoma and non-melanoma skin cancer, early childhood excessive sun exposure is an important risk factor for the development of skin cancer two or three decades later. This observation emphasizes the point that the development of cutaneous malignancy is a multistep process, and that one or more of the initial steps may occur very early in life. This clearly has implications for skin cancer prevention campaigns.

Exposure to ionizing radiation is an additional factor which predisposes to cutaneous malignancy, but modern methods of limiting such exposure makes this a relatively rare cause by comparison with exposure to ultraviolet radiation.

Similarly, although chemical carcinogens have been used traditionally in studies of cutaneous carcinogenesis using animal models, their role in the current epidemic of skin cancer in man appears small.

Benign cutaneous tumours

The differential diagnosis of a malignant cutaneous lesion will include a variety of benign skin tumours. In general, these are very much commoner than the malignant lesions and it is, therefore, important to be able to recognize these lesions.

Seborrhoeic keratoses (Basal cell papilloma, seborrhoeic wart)

Definition

A benign proliferation of epidermal keratinocytes.

Seborrhoeic keratoses are extremely common and become commoner with increasing age. Their aetiology is unknown, and despite the term seborrhoeic wart, the human papilloma virus does not appear to be a causative factor. Clinically,

Fig. 14.1 Classic basal cell papilloma. Note greasy warty surface and superficial stuck-on appearance in relation to the underlying skin.

Fig. 14.2 Flat type of seborrhoeic keratosis or basal cell papilloma on facial skin. This type of lesion can be confused with a lentigo maligna melanoma (p. 000).

they present as raised, frequently multiple lesions, mainly on covered body sites (Figs 14.1 and 14.2). Many are brown due to benign and incidental melanocytic activity within the lesion, and may therefore be mistaken for more serious problems such as malignant melanoma. The very superficial 'stuck on' appearance is a helpful differential point, and the keratin cysts are useful when making a clinical diagnosis, although there is a flat variant found on the face which may be difficult to distinguish from an early malignant melanoma (see below).

In lesions in which the diagnosis is clear-cut, removal is not essential. If removal is requested, curettage and diathermy is acceptable treatment, but the lesions are multiple and tend to recur.

Epidermal naevi

Definition

A raised, often linear plaque arising from a localized, benign proliferation of epidermal keratinocytes.

It is currently suggested that epidermal naevi arise as a result of an aberrant clone of keratinocytes. Epidermal naevi are relatively common, and range from a small raised area, often mistaken for a viral wart, to a very large and disfiguring pigmented area of hyperkeratosis covering 30 per cent of the body surface and associated with neurological problems. This is known as the epidermal naevus syndrome.

Epidermal naevi are not usually visible at birth but develop during childhood. Initially, there may just be an area of hyperpigmentation but over a period of months or years this becomes rough and hyperkeratotic. In flexural areas, this may result in bacterial colonization and secondary infection leading to discomfort. Many of these naevi are linear (Figs 14.3 and 14.4). Extreme and severe cases may be associated with systemic problems.

Fig. 14.3 Linear warty epidermal naevus on the trunk of a young man.

A variant of the epidermal naevus is the so-called **Becker's naevus** (Fig. 14.5) which is an area of faint hyperpigmentation and associated hypertrichosis. It is most commonly seen on the skin over the shoulder area, and may develop after sunburn.

Treatment of epidermal naevi is unsatisfactory. With small lesions no treatment may be necessary, and, with larger lesions, abrasion and keratolytics may reduce the hyperkeratosis. In some cases surgical excision is the most acceptable option.

Fig. 14.4 Extensive epidermal naevus covering a large part of one half of the body in an older boy.

Fig. 14.5 Becker's naevus. Note subtle pigmentation and some increase in hair growth over the shoulder area.

Pyogenic granuloma

Definition

A rapidly growing, benign tumour arising from the cutaneous vasculature.

Fig. 14.6 Pyogenic granuloma. Tender raised lesions develop over a period of 1–2 weeks.

Classically, these lesions develop after trauma, commonly on the fingers of keen gardeners after pruning roses (Fig. 14.6). Over a period of 2–3 weeks a raised, wet, pedunculated lesion develops and frequently becomes secondarily infected. The rapidity of growth may give rise to concern about a malignant lesion, but the natural history is of spontaneous regression over a period of weeks or months. The histological appearance is of a network of capillaries embedded in an oedematous stroma.

Surgical excision or diathermy is recommended as the lesions can be painful and inconvenient.

Histiocytoma (dermatofibroma, sclerosing angioma)

Definition

A firm flesh coloured nodule, most commonly on the lower leg.

This lesion appears most commonly as a firm, elevated nodule on the leg (Fig. 14.7). In some cases there is a history of trauma, such as an insect bite, to the site. The nodule is often brown and this pigmentation, together with a history of fairly rapid enlargement, may suggest that the lesion is a malignant melanoma. In fact, however, the pigment is chiefly iron rather than melanin and the lesion is quite benign.

Local excision may be necessary to obtain histological confirmation of the diagnosis.

Skin appendage tumours

Definition

A wide range of usually benign lesions arising from cells comprising the hair follicle, sebaceous glands, eccrine and apocrine sweat glands.

From the above definition it will be apparent that there is a very large range of tumours in this group, and discussion of them all is beyond the scope of this book, as many are very rare. Skin appendage tumours arise most commonly on the head and neck area and are clinically identified as small non-specific nodules. The usual preoperative diagnosis, if one is made, is of a basal cell carcinoma. The three skin appendage tumours most likely to be encountered in non-specialist practice are the organoid or sebaceous naevus, the pilomatricoma or calcifying epithelioma of Malherbe, and the eccrine poroma.

The **organoid or sebaceous naevus** is a localized area of excessive components of the pilosebaceous apparatus, usually of the sebaceous gland component (Fig. 14.8). They are seen clinically as raised, irregular, yellow nodules most commonly on the scalp and are often first seen in the first and second decades of life. Their importance lies in the fact that basal cell carcinoma may develop at an early age in between 10 and 25 per cent of these lesions. For this reason, prophylactic surgical removal with a narrow margin of normal skin is recommended.

The **pilomatricoma** is a common, benign tumour of childhood, and presents often in the first decade as a raised nodule on any part of the body surface. They are usually excised to obtain a histological diagnosis, and arise from the hair follicle.

The **eccrine poroma** arises from the eccrine sweat gland apparatus and is usually seen on older adults on the foot, presenting as a raised, red, moist nodule.

Some skin appendage tumours have malignant counterparts, but these are excessively rare. Local excision of the benign skin appendage tumours is usually necessary both to obtain a diagnosis and as a cure.

Premalignant lesions and carcinoma *in situ*

Actinic keratoses

Definition

Actinic keratoses are scaly, erythematous often irritable, hyperpigmented, crusting lesions, seen most often on the scalp, face, and back of the hands

Fig. 14.8 Organoid naevus on scalp. Note large yellowish papillomatus lesion.

Key Points

Premalignant lesions and carcinoma *in situ* should be identified and treated to prevent malignant change.

Fig. 14.9 Actinic keratosis on the face and hands of a male who has spent some time in the Tropics.

Fig. 14.10 Higher power view of multiple actinic keratoses on a male scalp.

(Figs 14.9 and 14.10). They are extremely common, and usually multiple, on the skin of fair skinned individuals who have enjoyed an outdoor occupation or recreation.

The striking histological changes in the epidermis are a loss of the normal keratinocyte maturation pattern, with some epidermal cells showing individual cell keratinization, and the appearance in the dermis of a dense area of 'elastic' tissue replacing the collagen of the papillary dermis—the so-called senile or actinic elastosis.

Actinic keratoses were commonest in the past on outdoor workers. Nowadays, however, recreational rather than occupational sun exposure is likely to be an important factor. Genetic factors are also important, and the fair- or red-haired, blue-eyed, freckled individual who tans poorly and burns easily is particularly at risk. Actinic keratoses have the potential for transformation into metastasizing squamous carcinoma. One Australian study has suggested that the rate of malignant transformation is around 1 per cent per year. However, most individuals have not only one but usually 10–20 actinic keratoses, and thus the risk of malignant change over time is higher. In practice, actinic keratoses should be treated because of the risk of malignant change, and patients should be given advice about sunscreen and hat use to reduce further sun exposure, as there is now good evidence that if such advice is taken that some of these actinic keratoses will regress.

Treatment

Treatment of existing actinic keratoses can be by cryotherapy, or topical application of the cytotoxic preparation 5-fluorouracil (Efudix). This preparation has the interesting property of 'seeking out' and stimulating an inflammatory esponse in 'preactinic' lesions which are not yet clinically visible. It is applied topically to the affected areas daily, carefully avoiding the eyes. After 2–3 weeks a brisk inflammatory reaction develops and the skin looks temporarily very much worse. After this, the lesions slowly clear with a good end-result.

If a lump or bump on the skin is worth removing in the surgery, it is worth sending for pathological reporting. In this way you will not make the tragic mistake of curetting off an early melanoma and arranging no further treatment.

Bowen's carcinoma *in situ* (Bowen's disease)

Definition

A form of intraepidermal carcinoma *in situ*, which on rare occasions progresses to invasive squamous carcinoma.

Clinical features

Clinically, Bowen's disease presents as an isolated, scaling, erythematous plaque, generally on the trunk (Fig. 14.11). It may look like an isolated patch of psoriasis and is frequently initially treated as such. If untreated, the lesions slowly expand laterally over a period of years and a very small proportion develop into metastasizing squamous carcinomas.

Pathology

The histological features include thickening of the epidermis (acanthosis) and lack of normal organization and maturation within the epidermis.

Treatment

Cryotherapy is a common and acceptable form of therapy. Many dermatologists first confirm their clinical diagnosis with an incisional biopsy.

Fig. 14.11 Scaling lesions of Bowen's disease on lower leg of elderly female.

Keratoacanthoma

Definition

A rapidly developing epidermal nodule with pathological features almost indistinguishable from squamous cell carcinoma.

Keratoacanthomas usually develop as raised solitary lesions on the face and may grow over 2–3 weeks to a size of 2–3 cm in diameter (Fig. 14.12). Thereafter, the nodule develops a necrotic, crusted centre, and clears spontaneously often leaving an unsightly pitted scar.

Fig. 14.12 Keratoacanthoma. This lesion had grown to the size seen in a period of 3–4 weeks.

Treatment

Currently, some pathologists are very reluctant to report a lesion as a keratoacanthoma because of the very real difficulty in differentiating it from a squamous cell carcinoma, and for both this reason and the risk of scarring, it is current practice to excise these lesions with a narrow margin of surrounding normal skin.

Cutaneous malignancies

Squamous cell carcinoma

Definition

A malignant tumour derived from keratinocytes.

The great majority of squamous carcinomas arise on sun-damaged skin. A few may develop in scar tissue. Squamous cell carcinomas are commoner on the sun exposed skin of transplant recipients, and the risk of developing squamous cell carcinoma increases with duration of transplant.

Clinical features

Clinically, the lesions present as hyperkeratotic, ulcerated, expanding nodules (Fig. 14.13). Metastatic spread to the local draining lymph nodes and beyond can occur.

Pathology

The striking histological features are gross disorganization of the epidermis with invasion of tongues of epidermal tissue and isolated discrete foci of neoplastic keratinocytes within the dermis. Mitotic figures, both normal and abnormal, are frequent.

Key Points

Basal cell carcinoma is the most common form of cutaneous malignancy.

Fig. 14.13 Invasive squamous carcinoma.

Treatment

Once a histological diagnosis has been established by biopsy, the tumour can be treated by excision or radiotherapy. In most centres surgical excision with an adequate margin of normal tissue is the preferred option. Patients should be on regular follow-up thereafter to detect recurrence.

Xeroderma pigmentosum

Definition

A group of genetically determined disorders associated with low levels of unscheduled DNA repair after exposure to ultraviolet radiation, and associated with a very high incidence of all types of cutaneous malignancy, particularly squamous cell carcinoma.

At present, at least five complementation groups (A to E) of xeroderma pigmentosum (XP) are recognized. The condition is inherited by autosomal recessive transmission, and the two commonest groups are A and C. Children in affected families show prolonged UV induced erythema in the first year of life, and this is quickly followed by grossly accelerated photoageing changes if the child is not protected from further sunlight exposure. Exposed skin becomes freckled, telangiectatic, and atrophic (Fig. 14.14), and before the age of five the child will have actinic keratoses, and squamous cell carcinoma. They are also at risk of developing basal cell carcinoma and malignant melanoma. Patients with XP groups A and B also have central nervous system degenerative problems.

Treatment

If a regime of total sun avoidance is practised, these children can grow to adult life.

Fig. 14.14 Xeroderma pigmentosum. Gross sun damage is seen on the facial skin of this 12-year-old girl.

Basal cell carcinoma (rodent ulcer)

Definition

A common, slowly growing, and locally destructive tumour thought to arise from a subset of the basal cells in the epidermis.

This tumour is by far the commonest form of cutaneous malignancy, but attracts less attention than squamous carcinoma or malignant melanoma.

Pathology

A mass of basophilic keratinocytes is seen pushing down into the dermis but retaining its contact with the overlying epidermis. Mitotic figures are plentiful but the turnover time is slow.

Clinical features

Basal cell carcinomas are seen predominantly on exposed sites, commonly around the nose and inner canthus. Initially, the lesion is a reddish, dome-shaped nodule with a translucent surface and visible, dilated surface capillaries. As it expands, the central area may show necrosis and ulceration, leaving the characteristic rolled edge (Fig. 14.15). The lesion has frequently been growing for 1–2 years before the patient seeks advice and further slow growth will continue if the lesion is not treated. Although these lesions do not metastasize, they may cause extensive and distressing local destruction of soft tissue, cartilage, and even bone (Fig. 14.16).

Treatment

Basal cell carcinoma can be treated either by surgery or by radiotherapy. In frail and elderly patients, curettage or cryotherapy may be acceptable therapy but

Fig. 14.16 Basal cell carcinoma.

Fig. 14.15 Basal cell carcinoma.

follow-up is essential. The prognosis is excellent and follow-up should be aimed at early detection of local recurrence, more common in certain sites, such as the nasolabial fold, and with certain morphoeic histological variants. In the very rare instances when a basal cell carcinoma is thought to metastasize the histology should be reviewed as the lesion may have been a tumour arising from one of the skin appendages.

In rare cases of recurrent basal cell carcinoma or **morphoeic basal cell carcinoma**, the tissue sparing technique of **Mohs surgery** can be very useful, particularly if the lesion is close to vital structures such as the eye. The principle behind this technique is to remove every single tumour cell but as little normal tissue as is necessary. Basically, the tumour is pared away in thin slices, and carefully oriented pathological examination is carried out on each slice.

A rare, genetically determined condition, **Gorlin's syndrome**, is characterized by the appearance of multiple basal cell carcinomas, jaw cysts, palmoplantar cutaneous pits, and skeletal abnormalities. Inheritance is by an autosomal dominant gene, now located to chromosome 9q31, and lesions are first seen in childhood. The basal cell carcinomas in this condition should be treated by surgery and not by radiotherapy as further new tumours may develop in the irradiated field.

Key Points

Remember to ask about tumour thickness for your melanoma patient. It has a very important bearing on prognosis.

Cutaneous malignant melanoma

Introduction

Malignant melanoma is probably the most important disease discussed in this book for three reasons:

1. The incidence is rising rapidly.
2. If identified and treated early, it is curable, but if not identified until a later growth stage, it is likely to cause the patients death.
3. A high proportion of melanoma patients are young adults.

Incidence and aetiology

At present there are about 10 new cases of melanoma per 100,000 of the population per year in Europe and the United States, but much higher numbers in Australia and New Zealand where the incidence is the highest in the world. The lifetime risk of developing melanoma in the UK at present is one in a hundred, but as the incidence is doubling in each decade, this figure is likely to become higher.

Numbers of melanoma cases are highest among the white skinned individuals in countries with long hours of strong sunshine. In addition to this observation, case control studies strongly suggest that exposure to sunlight is the major cause of melanoma. Emigrant studies looking at populations who emigrate from, for example, Europe to Australia or Israel as young children show that early childhood sun exposure is an important risk factor for melanoma in later life as adults.

Thus, exposure to natural UV appears to be the major risk factor for developing melanoma. Exposure to long-wave artificial UV from sunbed sources (UVA) appears also to be a risk factor.

However, some melanomas do develop on body sites rarely exposed to the sun, such as the sole of the foot, but at present no obvious causative factor other than UV exposure has been identified and confirmed for cutaneous malignant melanoma.

Genetics

An active search is in progress for the melanoma gene at the present time. Five per cent of melanomas are familial, and in a proportion of these familial melanoma cases genes in the area around chromosome 9p21 appear to be involved. The gene under most active current investigation is p16.

Pathology

Malignant melanocytes are seen to arise from melanocytes in the basal area of the epidermis and invade the underlying dermis. The depth to which these malignant cells have invaded is the most important prognostic factor for patients with primary melanoma. This measurement, which is made in millimetres, is called the tumour or **Breslow thickness** (Fig. 14.17). It is essential that the pathologist reporting melanoma includes this in his report as it is vital for prognosis for the individual patient. For example if an invasive malignant melanoma is less than 1 mm thick, there is an over 90 per cent chance that the patient will be alive and disease free at the end of 5 years, whereas if the tumour is thicker than 3 mm the likelihood of disease free survival falls to only 50 per cent.

Clinical features

Malignant melanoma is most commonly seen on the female leg and the male back in younger adults, and on the face in both sexes in older adults. At present, more females than males develop melanoma in the UK, but in most parts of the

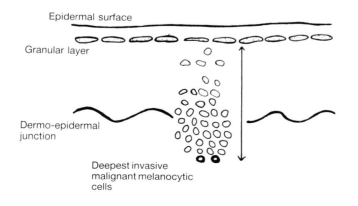

Malignant melanoma thickness measurement (Breslow)

Epidermal surface

Granular layer

Dermo-epidermal junction

Deepest invasive malignant melanocytic cells

Fig. 14.17 Diagrammatic representation of tumour thickness measured by the Breslow method. The distance between the granular layer and the deepest tumour cell (arrowed) is the Breslow thickness in millimetres.

world the incidence between the sexes is equal. Melanoma presents as a growing, changing area of pigmentation and the seven point check list may be useful in identifying early melanoma and differentiating it from other pigmented lesions.

The seven point checklist comprises three major signs:

1. change in shape
2. change in size
3. change in colour

and four minor signs:

4. over 5 mm in diameter
5. inflammation
6. crusting or bleeding
7. symptoms of minor itch or irritation.

Patients with lesions with one major and one or more minor signs should be considered for an excision diagnostic biopsy. The seven point checklist is sensitive but not specific, so that conditions other than cutaneous malignant melanoma may be included, but true melanoma is unlikely to be excluded.

Four subdivisions of melanoma can be recognized from clinical pathological grounds. The commonest of these is the **superficial spreading malignant melanoma** (Figs 14.18, 14.19, and 14.20) which comprises around 80 per cent of all melanomas in Caucasians. It is relatively easy to recognize as an irregularly shaped, expanding, pigmented lesion with more than one colour. Shades of brown, blue, or black are present. A rarer but more aggressive type is the **nodular melanoma** (Fig. 14.21) which is a rapidly growing red or black nodule on the skin with no surrounding pigmentation. Early bleeding is frequent. In older patients, the **lentigo maligna melanoma** variant is seen most often. This is the most slowly growing variety, and is usually seen on the face as a gradually

Fig. 14.18 Superficial spreading melanoma on inner malleolus area of female leg.

Fig. 14.19 High power view of superficial spreading melanoma showing irregularity in pigmentation.

Fig. 14.20 High power view of superficial spreading melanoma showing irregular margin.

Fig. 14.22 Lentigo maligna melanoma.

expanding flat lesion on the cheek (Fig. 14.22) which, if not treated, will develop raised central nodules over time. The rarest type of melanoma on Caucasian skin, but the commonest on Asian skin, is the **acral melanoma** found on the palms and soles (Fig. 14.23). This again is a slowly expanding, irregularly shaped area of pigmentation.

A variant of the acral melanoma is the **subungual melanoma**, found around the nail bed apparatus. This may present as an area of pigmentation on the nail or around the nail fold, but is frequently not recognized until it has partially destroyed the nail (Fig. 14.24).

Early melanoma is generally pain free, and the only symptom which patients complain of, if any, is of mild irritation or itch.

Fig. 14.21 Nodular melanoma.

Fig. 14.23 Acral melanoma.

Fig. 14.24 Subungual melanoma.

Differential diagnosis

The lesions to be included in the differential diagnosis of malignant melanoma include all types of benign melanocytic naevi and other non-melanocytic pigmented lesions such as seborrhoeic keratoses or even angiomas.

For superficial spreading malignant melanomas, the commonest differential diagnosis is between superficial spreading malignant melanoma and melanocytic naevi. The history of growth, the irregular outline, and the colour variation all suggest the lesion is likely to be melanoma rather than a naevus, as benign naevi are usually static in an adult, have a regular margin, and are composed of one shade of brown or black. For nodular malignant melanoma, the differential diagnosis may be between a vascular tumour or histiocytoma. This is the most difficult differential diagnosis and an excision biopsy is recommended if there is any clinical doubt.

For lentigo maligna melanoma a differential diagnosis is most commonly from the flat type of seborrhoeic keratosis or basal cell papilloma.

Treatment

If malignant melanoma is suspected a diagnostic excision biopsy with a narrow margin of normal skin should be performed without delay. The pathologist reporting the lesion should indicate the tumour thickness as on this will depend the future surgery. In the past decade it has become recognized that the extensive excisions previously practised for malignant melanoma were unnecessary. Although there is still some debate and ongoing research as to just how narrow the excision margins can be, a useful working measurement is to excise one centimetre of normal tissue around the malignant melanoma for every millimetre of thickness up to 3 cm. There is no evidence that a tumour margin greater than 3 cm confers any survival advantage on the patient. Thus, this means that nowadays many melanomas can be excised and the wound closed directly without grafting. It is important, however, to excise adequately in depth as well as in breadth.

As already stated, the patient's prognosis will depend on tumour thickness. For patients with tumours less than 1.5 mm, regular follow-up is all that is need, as the likelihood of recurrence is small. Indeed the risk of a second primary melanoma is greater in this group and the patient should, therefore, be examined carefully with this in mind. Patients with thicker tumours have a greater chance of recurrence, but there is as yet no proven method of preventing this. Patients with thick tumours, 3 mm or greater in depth, should be referred to a specialist centre for consideration for entering into trials of adjuvant therapy. Currently, there are many trials of adjuvant interferon therapy in progress, but as yet no evidence that this confers a survival advantage.

More advanced malignant melanoma, which has spread to the lymph nodes and to other organs in the body, should be treated in a specialist centre. Further surgery will be required, and patients may then enter into controlled trials of chemotherapy. Once melanoma has spread beyond the skin the prospects for survival are very poor.

Histiocytosis X

This is a rare proliferative disorder of the epidermal Langerhans cell. Opinion is divided as to whether it is a true malignancy or a hyperproliferative condition. Patients usually present as infants with a greasy rash on the scalp and in the flexures. This can look like severe seborrrhoeic dermatitis, but there is also hepatosplemomegaly.

Merkel cell carcinoma

Malignancies arising from the Merkel cell are also rare. They are usually found on the head and neck area of older people, and present as non-specific nodules. The treatment is surgery, but the prognosis is poor and about 50 per cent of patients develop metastatic spread.

Kaposi's sarcoma

This malignancy arising from the dermal endothelial cells has already been discussed in the context of AIDS. However, Kaposi's may also develop in non-HIV positive individuals, and is seen more commonly in those of Mediterranean origin, and in patients after chemotherapy.

Cutaneous lymphoma

A small number of lymphomas may actually arise in the skin or preferentially involve it. Most of these are demonstrated by membrane marker studies to originate from T lymphocytes.

Mycosis fungoides

Definition

A slowly evolving T cell lymphoma initially involving the skin.

Molecular biological studies of the T cell receptor gene rearrangements found in this condition suggest that this condition is clonal from an early stage in its evolution.

Pathology

The salient histological feature is the presence of a T cell lymphoid infiltrate in the papillary dermis and epidermis. These T cells are mainly T helper cells and are morphologically atypical.

Clinical features

The condition is seen mainly in middle-aged or elderly individuals who present with pruritic, cutaneous plaques (Fig. 14.25). They may involute spontaneously, remain relatively unchanged, or progress to frank nodules and ulceration

Key Points

Cutaneous lymphoma could be confused initially with psoriasis.

Figs 14.25 and 14.26 Cutaneous lymphoma of mycosis of fungoides type.

(Fig. 14.26). A small number of patients present with nodular lesions from the start and others present with poikiloderma (dappled skin)—a macular pigmentary change with alternating increased and decreased pigmentation.

The lesions are usually associated with severe and persistent pruritus.

Treatment

Treatment is aimed at control, rather than cure, of the disease. Topical steroids, conventional ultraviolet light (UVB), and photochemotherapy (PUVA) all improve symptoms; the latter may cause dramatic regression of lesions, but maintenance therapy is generally required. A course of electron beam therapy or low-penetration superficial X-rays may alleviate symptoms for long periods of time and are useful methods of therapy if the patient is unable to attend a centre for maintenance therapy. In general, mycosis fungoides responds poorly to systemic chemotherapy, but the regular use of topical nitrogen mustard is of value.

Metastases to the skin from tumours arising in other organs

Patients with advanced malignancy of any type may develop metastases to the skin, and very occasionally cutaneous metastases may be the first sign of such a malignancy. Breast tumours may metastasise to the scalp, causing painful nodules and hair loss. The diagnosis is made by biopsying the cutaneous nodule, and then initiating a careful search for the primary site.

Prevention of cutaneous malignancy

At the present time, cutaneous cancer is the commonest of all malignancies on a world-scale. Moreover, it is likely that the numbers of affected patients will increase with an ageing population and even greater sun exposure. This trend should be able to be partially prevented or reversed by encouraging safe and restricted sun exposure aimed at avoiding sunburn. This must begin early in life, and mothers should be asked to keep children out of midday sun, to use T-shirts and hats to protect the skin, and to use high SPF, broad spectrum sunscreens.

Discussion of problem cases

Case 14.1

While programmes such as the one described have a valuable educational role in encouraging self awareness about skin lesions and prompting earlier self referral with true skin malignancy, they also result in a large number of consultations from the 'worried well' who require reassurance. It is very useful to be able to triage these patients into those who have no serious problem and require only reassurance and an explanation of the nature of their lesion, those who have a possibly more serious problem and who require an excisional or incisional biopsy to obtain a tissue diagnosis, and those who do appear to have true cutaneous malignancy and require definitive treatment.

The description of the first patient suggests that she has several seborrhoeic keratoses or basal cell papillomas on her back. They are very common on the trunk of older, white skinned individuals, and have no premalignant potential. They frequently crumble or lose some substance after minor trauma, but tend to regrow, and may become quite large. No definitive treatment is necessary, unless a lesion is being irritated by clothing. Removal by curettage and cautery is normal treatment.

The second patient illustrates a relatively common problem with congenital melanocytic naevi. There is a very small risk of malignant change but minor, non-malignant, degenerative changes are much commoner. However, it is not usually possible to confidently differentiate between the two on clinical grounds, and pathological examination is needed. The young man had an excision biopsy with a margin of 2 mm of normal skin around the naevus. Pathological examination confirmed that the areas of increased pigmentation were due to benign proliferation within the naevus, and that there was no evidence of malignant change.

The third patient is the most worrying. Growing, changing, pigmented lesions in adults should be regarded with suspicion and this is the usual way in which cutaneous malignant melanoma presents. The irregular outline, and the fact that the lesion is multicoloured are additional worrying points. This lesion was excised with a margin of 5 mm of surrounding normal skin, and pathological examination confirmed that it was a superficial, spreading, malignant melanoma which was 0.48 mm thick and non-ulcerated, a good prognosis lesion. The scar was re-excised with 1 cm of normal skin in all directions, including in depth. Three years later she is well with no evidence of recurrence. What would you examine this patient for at follow up visits?

Case 14.2

This description suggests an area of Bowen's intraepidermal carcinoma *in situ*, an extrafacial basal cell carcinoma, or even an isolated patch of psoriasis, although solitary patches of psoriasis are extremely rare. The fact that he also has prostatic cancer is probably not relevant to this lesion, as although cutaneous metastases from prostate cancer do occur, they are commonly multiple nodules.

An excisional biopsy into the edge of the lesion confirmed that the plaque was an extrafacial basal cell carcinoma, and thereafter the entire plaque was excised with a narrow margin of surrounding normal skin and the wound closed directly.

Case 14.3

This patient clearly needs appropriate investigation to exclude remediable causes of hair loss including haematological and thyroid function assessment (p. 212). The nodule below her eye should be examined carefully. It is raised, translucent, and has visible capillaries on the surface. This picture strongly suggests basal cell carcinoma. An excision biopsy was therefore arranged, and pathological examination confirmed that the diagnosis was basal cell carcinoma, and that the lesion was completely excised. What follow up plans would be appropriate?

Case 14.4

This description and the outdoor occupation of the patient strongly suggests that the lesions are actinic keratoses. The fact that he is a fair skinned red head makes this even more likely. Multiple actinic keratoses can be treated by several methods including cryotherapy, or by the use of topical 5 fluorouracil (Efudix). This patient had three sessions of cryotherapy with obvious improvement. He was also advised to use a high SPF broad spectrum sunscreen throughout the year, and to wear a hat in sunny weather.

Projects

1. Review the current classifications of lymphoma and look at the place of cutaneous lymphoma. Are the current classification systems satisfactory for dermatologists?

2. Consider the likely impact of the ageing populations in the industrialized countries on non-melanoma skin cancer incidence figures. Are there any steps which could be taken that might change this?

Growth points

Dermatoscopy or epiluminescence

For many years, dermatologists in a hospital setting have used operation microscopes to try to improve their preoperative accuracy in diagnosing cutaneous melanoma. There are now inexpensive hand held machines available which may make this technique applicable in a wider setting. At present, the method requires critical audit, and it is obviously vital that no melanoma is incorrectly labelled a benign lesion.

Vaccine and gene therapy for melanoma

Melanoma is an immunogenic tumour, and a range of antigens which have relative, but not complete, specificity for melanoma have been identified. From these a wide range of vaccines have been developed which are now in clinical trials. They are most likely to be beneficial in patients who have a thick, primary tumour after removal of the lesion. Results are awaited.

Gene therapy is also available in a trial setting. The genes for interleukin 2 and for other biological response modifiers are being introduced into melanoma patients, in this case usually those with more advanced disease, in the anticipation that they may stimulate a more effective cytotoxic reaction against tumour cells. Again results are not yet available

Further reading

Burg, G. and Braun-Falco, O. (1983). *Cutaneous lymphomas*. Springer-Verlag, Berlin.

MacKie, R.M. (1995). *Skin cancer*, (2nd edn). Martin Dunitz, London.

A detailed and comprehensive account of all types of skin tumours.

15

*Brief notes on topical
therapy*

When prescribing topical therapy several points must be borne in mind.

1. The active ingredient must be prescribed in the appropriate vehicle or base.

2. Adequate quantities must be prescribed and applied. One application of cream or ointment for an adult to cover the whole body requires 20 g, one application to hands or face 2–4 g.

3. Instructions must be given to the patient concerning frequency and quantity of application. For some conditions, for example scabies in a large family, written instruction sheets will increase the likelihood of successful therapy.

Vehicles (bases)

A vehicle is defined as the (usually) inert carrier of the active ingredient. Vehicles are made up of liquids, greases, and powders in varying proportions according to the final consistency required. Thus, liquids alone may be used as **wet dressings** or **tinctures**, liquids and powders result in a shake **lotion** which is cooling and drying due to evaporation, grease alone is an **ointment**, and a grease and powder mixture results in a **paste**.

Lotions are used in acutely inflamed and moist exudative conditions. A useful preparation is ichthyol 1 per cent in calamine lotion BP. Lotions may be applied directly to the skin or on swabs or dressings which have been soaked in the lotion. In either case, frequent changing of dressings (for example every 4 hours) is necessary as otherwise the lotion will crust and cake.

Liniments are lotions with some additional oil which tends to prevent this crusting and it is therefore possible to change dressings less frequently. The advantage of rapid evaporation and cooling is, however, lost.

Creams

These are either oil-in-water or water-in-oil emulsions and contain preservatives to prevent bacterial and fungal growth. The commonest preservatives are chlorocresol and parabens. Either may cause sensitization and subsequent allergic contact dermatitis. Oil-in-water emulsions rub into the skin and are easily washed off. They are therefore very suitable for use on the face, but may have a drying effect on the skin. Water-in-oil emulsions are greasier. Less evaporation of water from the skin surface is possible through these preparations and they are therefore useful in conditions characterized by dryness and flaking. Water-in-oil emulsions are based either on petrolatum or on lanolin, which is a potential sensitizing agent.

Ointments

Ointments contain no water but are greases with the permissible addition of up to 40 per cent of powder by weight. A higher concentration of powder would change the consistency of the preparation to such an extent that it would be a paste. The lack of water in ointments renders the use of preservatives unnecessary, but emulsifying agents are frequently added to facilitate spreading. Ointments are useful in any condition characterized by dry skin (for example atopic dermatitis, chronic hand dermatitis). They are less easily washed off than creams.

Pastes

These are greases containing more than 40 per cent powder by weight. They are useful for dry surfaces but are very difficult to remove.

Current advances

Modern dermatopharmacology is a large and important section of the pharmaceutical industry. The current trend is to devise totally synthetic vehicles with a high degree of cosmetic acceptability and many preparations are now available which are neither ointments nor creams, but have some of the advantages (and possibly disadvantages) of both. The tendency to use lanolin less and to avoid preservatives where possible should, in time, lead to a decrease in the incidence of medicament-induced allergic contact dermatitis.

Fatty acid-propylene glycol bases (FAPG) are a newer and generally well-accepted type of vehicle.

For use on the scalp lotions or **gels** are acceptable. Creams, ointments, and pastes all lead to problems with removal. Gels are semi-colloids which liquefy on contact with the skin and are a common base for acne preparations.

• Some dermatologists adopt the practice of diluting a commercially available steroid preparation to minimize side-effects rather than prescribing an alternative weaker preparation. The two hazards of dilution are, first, inactivation of the active ingredients by use of an inappropriate and incompatible diluent, and, second, the risk of bacterial contamination during dilution. For these reasons, the widespread use of diluted steroids is not recommended without a pharmacy that has experience and understanding of this practice.

Emollients

Emollients are now available in many different forms, as bath additives, as soap substitutes, and as creams and ointment. They are of great value in the regular care of ageing skin, and of all the dry skin conditions, particularly the ichthyoses and atopic dermatitis. The pruritus which frequently accompanies dry skin conditions can be significantly relieved by emollients and the need for topical steroids can be greatly reduced. This is of particular value in the management of paediatric problems.

Patients differ in their response to emollient preparations and, for this reason, it is good practice to initially offer a range of five or six preparations, so that the patient can select those most effective and acceptable. It is common to find that one preparation is preferred for the body and another for the face.

Useful emollients include:

• **soap substitutes**: Liquid paraffin 50 per cent in white soft paraffin, emulsifying ointment BP, unguentum Merck;

- **bath additives**: Alpha-keri, Oilatum emollient, Balneum, Emulsiderm, Hydromol;
- **general purpose preparations**: aqueous cream BP, Oilatum cream, Diprobase.

Sunscreens

For dermatological use, a broad spectrum sunscreen with a sun protective factor of 15 or more is required. This sun protective factor measures the time by which sun exposure can be increased before any reddening of the skin occurs by comparison with non-protected skin. Sunscreens contain both chemical and physical sunscreens. In general, the physical agents, such as microfine titanium dioxide, are the most effective but may not be as cosmetically acceptable. Effective preparations include Sun E45, Spectraban 15 lotion, Roc 15 A + B cream, and Coppertone Supershade 15.

Topical steroid preparations

Topical steroid has already been discussed in the relevant treatment sections, and their undesirable side-effects in Chapter 12.

It is good practice to use regularly only one or two topical steroids from each potency group and to be aware of the value of increasing and decreasing steroid potencies as the condition indicates.

The choice of dressing

The need for frequent renewal of topical preparations is reduced by the use of appropriate dressings. For trunk and limbs expandable stockinet dressings can be made into neatly fitting 'body suits' and worn under normal clothing. Smaller areas can be covered with narrower dressings of similar material. When pastes are used it is often of value to spread the paste on to a dressing with a spatula and then apply the dressing to the area and bandage it in position. Large raw areas should be covered with a dressing such as sterile paraffin gauze which does not stick to the granulating surface.

In chronic dermatitis the use of occlusive tar or ichthyol impregnated bandages may help to break the itch-scratch-itch cycle and allow the skin to heal. These bandages (for example Coltapaste, Tarband, Ichthopaste) can be covered with a stockinet dressing and left in position for up to a week.

Occlusive dressings of this type are also extremely useful in the out-patient management of stasis ulcers. A dry gauze swab can be used to cover the ulcerated area and an Ichthopaste or Viscopaste bandage applied from the ankle to below the knee and covered with an elastocrepe bandage. This can be changed by the district nurse at weekly intervals or even less frequently. The Viscopaste bandages have the advantage of being easily unwound from the leg, even after 2–3 weeks in position.

Further reading

Bickers, D. R., Hazen, P. G., and Lynch, W. S. (1984). *Clinical pharmacology of skin disease*, Monographs in Clinical Pharmacology, Vol. 7. Churchill Livingstone, New York.

Seville, R. and Martin, E. (1981). *Dermatological nursing and therapy*. Blackwell Scientific Publications, Oxford.

A useful, inexpensive paperback.

Stone, L. A., Lindfield, E. M., and Robertson, S. (1989). A *colour atlas of nursing procedures in skin disorders*. Wolfe Medical Publications, London.

Reference sources

The two major English language textbooks currently available are:

1. Rook, A., Wilkinson, D. S. and Ebling, F.G.J. (ed.) (1992) *Textbook of dermatology*, (5th edn). (4 vols). Blackwell Scientific Publications, Oxford.

2. Fitzpatrick, T. B., Eisen, A. Z., Wolff, K., Freedberg, I.M., and Austen, K. F. (ed.) (1993) *Dermatology in general medicine*, (4th edn). McGraw-Hill; New York.

Both are very comprehensive but be sure you consult the most up-to-date edition.

A smaller, one volume book which is also useful is Braun-Falco, O., Plewig, G., Wolff, H. and Winkleman, R. (1990) *Dermatology*, Springer, Berlin.

A useful text on paediatric dermatology is Hurwitz, S. (1993) *Clinical Paediatric Dermatology*, (2nd edn). Saunders, Philadelphia.

When reviewing the literature it is useful to known the journals which are most likely to be helpful. The **Journal of the American Academy of Dermatology** has excellent review articles with many references and is well worth consulting.

Three of the general clinical journals well worth consulting are the **British Journal of Dermatology, Clinical and Experimental Dermatology** and the **American Archives of Dermatology**.

If you are more interested in experimental and investigative dermatology, then you should look for the **Journal of Investigative Dermatology**.

Index